Stop Gambling
for Good

Stop Gambling
for Good

Overcome Reckless Risk Taking with
Dr. Prasad's Proven Program

Balasa L. Prasad, M.D.

with Catherine Whitney

Avery   a member of Penguin Group (USA) Inc.   New York

Published by the Penguin Group
Penguin Group (USA) Inc., 375 Hudson Street, New York, New York 10014, USA •
Penguin Group (Canada), 90 Eglinton Avenue East, Suite 700, Toronto, Ontario M4P 2Y3,
Canada (a division of Pearson Penguin Canada Inc.) • Penguin Books Ltd, 80 Strand,
London WC2R 0RL, England • Penguin Ireland, 25 St Stephen's Green, Dublin 2, Ireland
(a division of Penguin Books Ltd) • Penguin Group (Australia), 250 Camberwell Road,
Camberwell, Victoria 3124, Australia (a division of Pearson Australia Group Pty Ltd) •
Penguin Books India Pvt Ltd, 11 Community Centre, Panchsheel Park, New Delhi–110 017,
India • Penguin Group (NZ), Cnr Airborne and Rosedale Roads, Albany, Auckland 1310, New
Zealand (a division of Pearson New Zealand Ltd) • Penguin Books (South Africa) (Pty) Ltd,
24 Sturdee Avenue, Rosebank, Johannesburg 2196, South Africa

Penguin Books Ltd, Registered Offices: 80 Strand, London WC2R 0RL, England

Library of Congress Cataloging-in-Publication Data

Prasad, Balasa.
Stop gambling for good: overcome reckless risk taking with Dr. Prasad's
proven program / Balasa L. Prasad with Catherine Whitney.
p.   cm.
Includes index.
ISBN 1-58333-235-9
1. Compulsive behavior. 2. Gambling. 3. Compulsion (Psychology).
I. Whitney, Catherine. II. Title.
RC569.5.G35P73   2005   2005047819
616.85'841—dc22

Printed in the United States of America
1   3   5   7   9   10   8   6   4   2

Book design by Meighan Cavanaugh

Neither the authors nor the publisher are engaged in rendering professional advice or services to the individual reader. The ideas, procedures, and suggestions in this book are not intended as a substitute for consulting a physician. All matters regarding health require medical supervision. Neither the authors nor the publisher shall be liable or responsible for any loss, injury, or damage allegedly arising from any information or suggestion in this book. The opinions expressed in this book represent the personal views of the authors and not of the publisher.

Most Avery books are available at special quantity discounts for bulk purchase for sales promotions, premiums, fund-raising, and educational needs. Special books or book excerpts also can be created to fit specific needs. For details, write Penguin Group (USA) Inc. Special Markets, 375 Hudson Street, New York, NY 10014.

While the authors have made every effort to provide accurate telephone numbers and Internet addresses at the time of publication, neither the publisher nor the authors assume any responsibility for errors, or for changes that occur after publication. Further, the publisher does not have any control over and does not assume any responsibility for author or third-party websites or their content.

This book is dedicated with love and gratitude to:

My parents, especially my mother. She was an extraordinary woman who instilled in me discipline, compassion, and a deep sense of responsibility. She taught me to dream big and work hard to make that dream a reality. She encouraged me to believe in myself and to do the best I could with my God-given talents.

My wife, Vashanta, who is the love of my life. She has always been a great inspiration for me—highly supportive, constantly encouraging me to work hard and to be proud of everything I do in my profession. She truly is a life partner at home and at work.

My daughter and only child, Bindu, a smart, wonderful young lady who has been my greatest fan and best critic. Bindu has always helped me with remarkable comments and suggestions.

They say that there is a woman behind every successful man, but in my case I feel blessed to have three smart and intuitive women who have helped me come this far in life.

ACKNOWLEDGMENTS

Special thanks to Judge Judy Sheindlin. When I was almost finished with my manuscript, I met Judge Judy who took a look at it and felt that it had great potential and put me in touch with her publishing agent immediately. I was excited because I have a great deal of respect for Judy. She is one of the most intelligent and astute individuals that I have had the pleasure of meeting. Judy's husband, Judge Gerald Sheindlin, has also been very helpful.

Endless thanks to Catherine Whitney, who thoroughly understood my philosophical and scientific approach in dealing with habits. She literally transformed my manuscript into an interesting and enlightening book. She is a wonderful writer, and I feel very lucky to have had the opportunity to work with her.

My thanks to my literary agents, Jane Dystel and Miriam Goderich, who took an early interest in my manuscript and believed in me. They worked tirelessly to see that my book found the right publishing home.

My editors at Avery/Penguin, Megan Newman and Kristen Jennings, have showed enthusiasm and creativity, and I am proud to have them behind my work. It was Megan who decided to present the material in a series of practical books in order to spread their impact as far as possible. Kristen has shepherded the manuscripts through the process with great sensitivity to my intentions.

Thanks to Dr. Preetham Grandhi, a child and adolescent psychiatrist, who engaged me in a healthy debate about psychiatric views. I am also grateful to the nursing staff at Mount Vernon Hospital in New York, who served as my spokespeople to my patients and the public. They are, and will always be, my biggest cheerleaders.

Last but not least, I want to thank my patients of the past twenty-five years, who have helped me to strengthen my beliefs and my profound philosophy. They have taught me firsthand that there are no simple answers to life's complex problems. It is very gratifying for me to know that I have been of help to them in dealing with challenges in their day-to-day life and that I have played a part in their happiness, health, and success.

CONTENTS

INTRODUCTION

The Slippery Slope

GAMBLING IS AS OLD as recorded history. Primitive peoples cast bones or sticks, in the same way that we throw dice. Ancient Rome held chariot races, the precursors to modern horse racing. Lotteries were used in the Middle Ages to pay war debts and build public works. In many Eastern societies, gambling has a long, revered history. There are reports that gambling was so common in China during the late nineteenth century that people regularly wagered with vendors for food and basic necessities, willing to risk going without a meal for the chance to win three meals.

Gambling has become one of the most popular forms of entertainment in America today. There are millions of recreational gamblers, who enjoy an occasional game of chance. Once in a while they like a change of pace, and gambling feels like a fun adventure. They get a slight thrill from the momentary uncertainty, but they're willing to take the chance because, for them, the stakes are not high. They're elated when they win, but not too devastated when they lose. They view it as the price of admission to an environment that provides more than just the games. Most casinos are located in attractive places that include excellent nightclubs, shows, restaurants, and shopping malls.

Recreational gamblers usually bet with their minds, not their hearts. They invariably operate on a predetermined budget plan. Most of them walk out once the allocated funds are exhausted. They rarely lose control. They rarely cross the safety limits. The key characteristic of recreational gamblers is their sense of control. They are not swept away by the thrill of risk taking. They do not deceive themselves. The illusion of winning big is perfectly balanced by the reality of losing big.

Even people who go to casinos regularly can be responsible gamblers. When I was visiting the casinos in Atlantic City to observe gambling behavior, one particular group of gamblers caught my attention: the elderly women, clutching plastic cups full of coins, pulling the levers of slot machines. They were deeply engrossed in this activity, only occasionally glancing at one another or their surroundings. I was amazed at their concentration, which sometimes lasted for hours without a break. I saw one woman playing three slot machines at the same time. Another woman played one slot machine for a short period, then moved to another, repeating this pattern every few minutes.

I watched them play, observing smiles and cries of delight when the machine poured out coins, and frowns when the machines were unresponsive. When one of the women decided to take a break from her gambling activities, I introduced myself and asked if I could buy her coffee. She agreed, and in exchange she told me about herself and her friends.

Her name was Shirley. She said that most of the elderly women in that casino were retired and lived alone. The majority of them were widowed, a few were divorced, and some had never been married. They were all on fixed incomes. Shirley said they came to the casino to escape the monotony of their lives. It could be boring and lonely to stay put and fix home-cooked meals day after day. I asked if they came for the companionship, and Shirley said, "Not really. I mean, we're not friends. It's nice to have other people around, but we don't socialize."

I guessed that these women were basically loners, and to some extent introverts. It was easy for them to hop on the bus to Atlantic City and engage in a personal relationship with the one-arm bandits. Shirley admitted that eventually everyone loses money to casinos, but if they play with some strategy, they can play longer and sometimes win a few bucks.

"We enjoy it—win or lose," she said. Maybe they were small-time compulsive gamblers, and maybe their activities weren't completely healthy, but Shirley justified it this way: "Instead of wasting money on psychologists, psychotherapists, and antidepressants, we come here and spend our money on the machines. It's comforting. Is that wrong?"

I smiled at Shirley, and told her I wouldn't presume to judge, but it was probably a harmless therapy for most of them. She nodded with satisfaction. "Just what I thought," she said, and stood up to return to her machine.

One striking difference between these women and the reckless, compulsive gambler is that the women knew what they were doing and why they were doing it. They set limits and had their fun, without expectation of magical rewards. Reckless, compulsive gamblers live in a bubble of illusion. They boast about their wins, but they resist facing their losses. They sit around, retelling the story of some big win that might have happened years earlier, even as their circumstances worsen. They're convinced that one of these days they'll have another big win that will solve all of their problems.

People have different views on where to draw the line between recreation and what they consider a taboo or potentially dangerous form of gambling. I've asked many people their views on gambling through the years. Lynn, a nurse, shrugged her shoulders in dismissal when I talked to her. "I don't gamble," she said. "I'm a sore loser. I'd rather spend my hard-earned money on the things I need. If any is left over, I put it in savings."

Lynn went on to say that she considered gambling a serious sickness and equated it to alcoholism or drug addiction. She concluded that gambling has no redeeming value. She would erase the word *gambling* from the dictionary if she could.

I responded that she could erase the word from the vocabulary but not the concept from the mind, because nature has written gambling in the human mind in indelible ink. "Haven't you ever purchased a lottery ticket?" I asked.

"Well, yes, once in a while when there's a big jackpot," Lynn acknowledged. "But I hardly call that *gambling*."

"You don't have to steal a million dollars to be called a thief," I said, teasing her a little. "A loaf of bread is enough." She got my point, but she still didn't consider a wager of a dollar or two comparable to gambling.

I also asked Peggy, a nurse's aide, what she thought about gambling, and she said she viewed herself as a sensible gambler. She set aside $5 a week for lottery tickets. She considered it recreation. Hope in the possibility of a jackpot made her feel good, and she didn't think $5 a week was too much to spend.

"This is something I've thought about," she said, "because my aunt, who died twenty years ago, was hooked on the numbers game. Everyone in the family knew about Aunt Rebecca. Each day, rain or shine, she walked down to the corner deli and played the numbers. Then she'd go home and spend the rest of the day planning which numbers she'd pick next. Gambling was her all-consuming passion.

"Once, when she was rushed to the hospital with severe abdominal pain, all she could think about was making her bet," Peggy recalled. "I was a teenager then, and as they were wheeling her out, she asked me to go to the deli and play her numbers. My mom wouldn't let me, and Aunt Rebecca was really mad."

"Do you think your aunt was addicted to gambling?" I asked.

Peggy thought about it for a moment, then replied, "She never lost very much money, but I'd have to say she was an addict because playing the numbers ruled her life." Peggy hit the nail on the head with her observation. It is the compulsion to gamble, not the amount you wager, or whether you win or lose, that determines if you have a gambling problem. These signs are merely the physical manifestations of the addiction. For this reason, it is possible to gamble recreationally without getting swept into an addictive cycle.

But for many people, gambling is a form of enslavement that robs them of everything they hold dear in life and drives them to the point of despair. There is hope for these addicted gamblers, and the program in this book is designed to help even those who have failed to quit in the past.

In this book I also address another form of reckless gambling—the drive that leads people to become "shopaholics" or credit card junkies. You will see that reckless spending is just another form of addictive gambling.

During the twenty-five years I've worked to help people overcome destructive habits that run the gamut from gambling to smoking to drug abuse to obsessive food cravings to sexual excess, I have witnessed remarkable transformations thousands of times. I am not saying that it is easy to give up the addictive pleasure that is so much a part of your life. The process requires strength and determination. I will help you discover that freedom holds a greater thrill than addiction.

The six steps of this program involve a focus on the mind of a pathological gambler, not on the gambling activity. The activity of gambling is merely a physical manifestation of a deeper craving triggered by the emotional center of the mind. When you liberate yourself from the mental slavery, you can experience a full and satisfying life, free from your addiction.

Part One

The Gambler's Mind

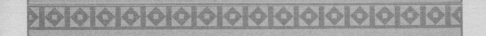

1

Life Is a Gamble

MOST PEOPLE consider gambling a somewhat unsavory activity. It brings to mind images of decadent casinos or sleazy back rooms where desperate players huddle around game tables as scantily clad waitresses supply them with unlimited alcoholic beverages. Gamblers are often portrayed in films and on TV as hapless fools swept up in an unhealthy fever. Paradoxically, as a nation we spend nearly $60 billion a year on games of chance. We constantly send a mixed message. More than two-thirds of our states have lotteries; there are off-track betting (OTB) outlets everywhere; and the number of casinos is on the rise. The Internet has added an entirely new landscape of chance. For the reckless, compulsive gambler, this easy availability of gambling is a recipe for disaster.

Humans are social animals, so most of us are constrained by cultural standards from behaving recklessly. But when we legalize gambling, license casino operators, and become reliant on lotteries to fund state programs, we not only eliminate the stigma, we actually encourage the behavior.

I'm not saying that the availability of gambling *creates* the addiction. However, every human being is born with the potential to become an addict because we are inherently pleasure seekers. If you eliminate the constant fear for survival, which we have effectively done in most modern societies, the pursuit of pleasure becomes dominant. For those who are so inclined, pleasure seeking becomes addictive. Society cannot refuse all responsibility in these matters.

Reckless, compulsive gambling is not just about money. It is about an entire series of behaviors—lying, cheating, stealing, self-deception, manipulation—that destroys families, betrays friendships, and ultimately leaves those afflicted with nothing to show for their lives.

George, a fifty-five-year-old mechanic, came to me for help with his gambling problem. Things were pretty bleak for George. His wife had left him the year before, his children refused to speak to him, and he was deeply in debt. Like many compulsive gamblers I've met over the years, George said he didn't really realize the severity of his problem until things had gone too far.

George couldn't believe he'd got himself into this mess because he'd always been a straight shooter, a guy who played by the rules. He'd never missed a day's work and he was devoted to his family. In fact, he'd started gambling because he wanted to give them a more comfortable life.

Several years earlier, George had started going to an OTB parlor on payday. Money was tight, but he thought it was worth taking a shot to gamble a few dollars. He dreamed of scoring big, and imagined himself surprising his wife, Bonnie, and his kids with the news that they'd never have to worry about money again. Over time, the amount of money George allotted for gambling increased, and he found himself thinking about the OTB parlor all week at work. He couldn't wait to grab his paycheck and head over there.

For a long time, George's wife had no idea that he was gambling. His wins and losses were so insignificant that they didn't affect their family life. But as George got bolder and, consequently, began to lose more, he could no longer keep his gambling secret. The shocks began to come, one after the other. "First it was the credit cards," he said. "Bonnie started getting calls from the collectors because the cards were maxed out and I couldn't make the payments. Next it was the house. I'd taken out a second mortgage, but I was having trouble making that payment, too. Basically, in a year's time I lost everything."

George's wife was so stunned by her husband's secret life, and so devastated by his betrayal, that she took the kids and left him. He didn't think she'd ever come back. "I really blew it," he said. "The crazy thing is, some part of me still thinks I can make it all up to her by a big win."

But don't be deceived into thinking that gambling is only a problem for losers. Take William J. Bennett, former government official and author of *The Book of Virtues*. Bennett has been called the conscience of our nation—a crusader for high moral standards. But recently it was revealed that for many years Bennett was a high-stakes gambler, with credit lines of at least $200,000 at several casinos in Atlantic City and Las Vegas. According to the *Washington Monthly*, he has lost more than $8 million over the years.

When his gambling habit became public, Bennett did not acknowledge that he had a problem. He did not express shame. Instead, he went on the offensive. He claimed he was not like those other pathetic compulsive gamblers who risked everything. He may have lost millions, but it was money he could afford to lose. He famously stated, "I never bet the milk money."

I'll leave it to others to evaluate the morality of Bennett's expensive habit. My interest is his compulsion to gamble. I believe that Bennett can be classified as a compulsive, reckless gambler. The fact that he has not yet lost everything is completely irrelevant. The key factor is the thrill he derives from playing big stakes and the sense of invincibility he possesses that he will never be overwhelmed by his habit. Sometimes so-called sensible compulsive gamblers are overconfident that their futures will not be affected by their compulsions. But they are no less slaves to their addictions than the perennial losers.

Michael was a case in point. He came to see me because of a gambling problem, but on the face of it Michael was in pretty good shape. At thirty-nine he had achieved success in business and he had a very nice lifestyle. He had a winning personality and a handsome, open face. But he was consumed by his gambling habit, sometimes playing poker three or four days at a stretch with his friends. Michael was single, and he knew if he wanted to get married and have children, he'd have to deal with his habit.

Michael told me that he'd loved gambling even as a teenager. He enjoyed the challenge of toying with the odds to work in his favor. For him gambling was a form of relaxation, a way to escape reality. His eyes sparkled as he described the pleasure he got from poker. "When I play, the outside world doesn't exist," he said. "Only the game. I concentrate completely. I love the feeling that I can control the result. Sometimes I get goose bumps, especially when I fake out my partners with a weak hand and win."

Michael did not drink alcohol or use drugs that would cloud

his judgment during a game. He always made sure to keep his mind clear and sharp while he played poker. The appeal of this particular game, as opposed to craps or roulette, was the feeling it gave Michael that he was betting on his skills, not just on chance. In fact, when he played poker, Michael believed he was actually betting on himself. And he usually won.

There was no question that Michael was a compulsive gambler, yet he was also a sensible gambler. He wasn't in debt, his judgment was clear, and he had the skills to win. His job and his lifestyle were not in jeopardy. I asked him the obvious question: "If playing poker is not a threat to your security, why have you come to see me?"

Michael's answer intrigued me. He said that although he had learned to master the technical aspects of the game, he could not control the emotional entanglement. He viewed his habit as ultimately irresponsible and childish. He was sick and tired of the emotional roller-coaster ride of a gambler's life. Lately, he had been thinking of getting married to his longtime girlfriend and he knew he'd have to make changes, but he wasn't sure he could give up the habit on his own. "Sometimes I feel like a slave to poker," he said honestly.

As we continued to talk, I learned that Michael's gambling control was not as great as he had implied. Beneath the surface, he was full of anxiety and fear. He admitted that although he won more than he lost, he'd lost plenty of money over the years. He'd thrown good money away—an intolerable scenario for a responsible husband and father.

"Wait a minute," I said. "I thought you told me your gambling wasn't posing a financial threat."

"It's not so much a matter of debt as it is of control," Michael said. He explained that he had great composure as long as he was winning. However, he was a sensitive, sore loser. He would lose control at a time when he was supposed to maintain a cool composure and bet with his head. When he was on a losing streak, he would bet recklessly and get even more upset. If he lost one hand, he'd become more impulsive on the next hand. "I am the gentle Dr. Jekyl when I'm winning and the nasty Mr. Hyde when I'm losing," he said with an embarrassed laugh.

Another problem Michael faced was the credit extension offered to players by the game organizers. In his opinion, when gamblers played with their own money, to some extent they were cautious. But once a gambler got into credit-line betting, there was no way that he could keep track of his losses. Michael also acknowledged that he had another weakness. He had no respect for his gambling gains. He always squandered his money on useless things. He never saved his gains to cover his losses. He told me that gambling was draining his spirit.

I was able to help Michael because he understood that the stakes were his very peace of mind and dignity. He did not have the illusion that gambling was a problem only when he lost money. He saw the larger picture—that the compulsion itself was robbing him of his freedom and corrupting his spirit.

Michael's case was unusual. Normally, compulsive gamblers who seek my help are in dire straits. They've hit rock bottom. They are unable to see their plight clearly, even in the face of disaster. Often they have associated addictions to alcohol or drugs, which further erode their clarity. For them, the endgame is truly a rock-bottom scenario, involving the destruction of their families, the loss of their jobs, and in some cases even incarceration.

George and Michael were very different gamblers—one had lost control over his habit and his life, while the other had not yet reached a point of crisis. But they both had unhealthy compulsions and I knew I could help them. When I met each of them, I began by making them understand one thing: you cannot *stop* gambling.

It's very simple. To be a human being, alive in the world, is to be a gambler. You cannot know what will happen to you in the next second or minute or week or year. Your life is a game of chance, and you are required to play it. The problem is not gambling itself, but the addictive compulsion to gamble recklessly. This distinction is an essential part of my philosophy when treating compulsive gamblers. They are so caught up in their phantasmagoric ideas that they've lost the ability to see the clear reality of human existence—*that life itself is a gamble.*

Nature demands that we gamble at all times on all occasions without hesitation. But nature also warns us that we must be sensible and smart about it—that we must perform a perfect balancing act on a very narrow bar where there is no room for error and no safety net. The setup has not changed throughout human history, and it will not change in the future. It is incumbent upon us to grin and bear it, and to accept nature's challenge in its entirety. Here's the bottom line: we will perish if we gamble too recklessly, and we will perish if we refuse to gamble at all. We are up against a rock and a hard place when it comes to our future, because every action we take, or fail to take, has definite consequences. What everyone must learn is how to handle the gambling instinct to our advantage and be savvy gamblers.

As I was studying the characteristics of the gambling instinct, I came upon a very interesting observation. There exists a close connection and a strong similarity between compulsive gambling and obsessive eating habits. Nature expects us to eat to survive. An obese individual cannot stop eating altogether to lose weight.

To manage proper healthy weight, he must keep tabs on what, when, where, and how much he eats. That is the reason it is an extremely tough task to maintain proper weight. We have no choice but to be smart and sensible about our eating habits. Gambling is in the same league. Every minute of the future is unknown, and we are required to choose an action—to go or stay, to drive or walk, to work or relax, to spend or save. *Webster's Dictionary* defines gambling as "an act that depends on chance, risk, or an uncertain venture." That's a pretty good description of life!

Consider how compulsions to overeat or gamble contrast with addictions to cigarettes, alcohol, or drugs. These substances are not necessary for survival. Once an individual recognizes that it is not in his best interest to pursue them, he can walk away without doing any harm to himself. Yet eating and gambling are governed by our instincts, meaning that they are connected to our very survival. Thus, disorders related to them must be managed differently.

The most perplexing thing about compulsive gambling, which has puzzled every expert, is the absence of a mind-altering chemical substance as a mediator in shaping this addiction. With addictions to alcohol, cigarettes, or drugs, we can identify a chemical substance and trace its effects on the development of an addiction. The absence of a physical medium to initiate the gambling addiction has made it tougher to classify it as a disease, but in my opinion this addiction is not that different from others. Chemical substances are merely triggers. The real problem is in the mind, not the substance or activity.

2

A Problem of the Mind,
Not the Brain

COMPULSIVE GAMBLING, like every addiction, is a problem of the mind, not the brain. The need or compulsion to engage with an addiction and the need to follow it through with an addictive activity are triggered by the mind and certainly not by the biological need of the brain or the body. This is true for all types of addiction, especially in the early stages. However, the addict is usually completely unaware that his emotional justifications are driving the addiction, not the activity itself.

As any person enslaved by a bad habit will tell you, it is not enough to know intellectually that something is bad for you and should be stopped. Most of my patients are completely baffled by their inability to respond to the most persuasive arguments about the harm their behavior is causing to their health, relationships, careers, and well-being. The reason for this disconnection lies in the complex nature of the mind, which involves the dynamic interplay of three divisions—intellect, emotions, and instinct.

The Intellectual, Emotional, and Instinctual Divisions of the Mind

The Intellectual Division of the mind receives information, then presents it to the Emotional Division for acceptance. The Emotional Division is the real policy maker, the one that calls the shots. When an individual can't break a habit, it is because the Intellectual Division has failed to make its case for giving up the habit to the Emotional Division, which says, "Sorry, I'm not convinced. This behavior feels good to me." Without the support of the Emotional Division, both the Intellect, which executes proper actions to safeguard the individual, and the Instincts, which control habitual behavior, are incapable of making short- or long-term corrections. The only argument the Emotional Division would accept at this point would be a radical one, such as, "The next time you pull the lever of the slot machine, you die." This is not realistic and therefore cannot be used as a convincing argument by the Intellect.

The human mind is a most effective, complex, and mysterious entity. It is capable of devising swift, savvy, and ingenious maneuvers to help us survive a harsh and ever-changing world. The mind, whose job it is to protect the interests of the individual, attempts to manipulate environmental forces to its advantage. When it fails to do so, it has no choice but to adapt grudgingly to the environmental requirements in order to survive. Unfortunately, when the environment and the mind do not see eye to eye, the mind suffers the stress of being out of sync with reality. So the mind has an extremely difficult assignment, with little room for error. Let's examine the interplay among the three divisions to better grasp these complex dynamics.

THE INTELLECTUAL DIVISION

The Intellectual Division harbors the pragmatic component of the mind, which we know as human intelligence. The individual characteristics of this intelligence are reasoning, judgment, logic, discretion, calculation, imagination, analysis, and anticipation. By virtue of these segments, the Intellectual Division is also known as the rational division of the human mind. It is the most complex, sophisticated and highly evolved section of the mind. Each and every component of the Intellectual Division exhibits a unique natural gift of its own which comes in handy in fulfilling this division's responsibility. Its responsibility is to absorb and analyze the barrage of information it receives from the environment, and to program an appropriate response. It appears that nature has picked each and every one of these components for its distinct talent, and purposefully grouped them together under one banner. This ingenious assortment of incredible characters has boosted the Intellectual Division into the front lines of our struggle for survival.

Utilizing the services of our five senses—sight, smell, hearing, taste, and touch—the Intellectual Division receives a steady stream of divergent messages and information from the environment. The individual components of the Intellectual Division analyze millions of bits of information and prepare an appropriate response. If the input from the environment is processed in the Intellectual Division without any interference or influence from the Emotional Division, the outcome of its analysis would be uniform and universal for everyone. Thus, despite each person having a diversified ethnic as well as geographic background, one would expect a stereotyped response to the environment from every human being of similar intellectual caliber. But in reality this is not the case. No two human beings are alike. They do not think the same way or have the same interests. Different human beings see the same set of facts from different perspectives. This diversity is caused primarily by the influence of the Emotional Division.

THE EMOTIONAL DIVISION

The Emotional Division, which I consider to be the most important, conscious counterpart of the Intellectual Division, accommodates two sets of powerful emotions—primitive and advanced. Primitive emotions are anger, rage, pain, pleasure, comfort, thrill, fear, fright, and selfishness. These primitive emotions are shared by almost all larger (macroscopic) terrestrial organisms. Advanced emotions are love, caring, affection, passion, compassion, concern, grief, deceit, jealousy, hate, greed, pride, and prejudice. The advanced emotions are shared by animal species of a higher intellectual order. The type and the number of advanced emotions are determined by the level of intelligence of the animal species. Human beings are the sole possessors of all levels of emotions, but the primitive emotions often remain the most potent. Love, affection, compassion, and concern are very refined and usually take a back seat to all others. They tend to lose out in an argument to more powerful, primitive emotions and to their close allies—jealousy, greed, hate, and vengeance. This fact is most evident in the human propensity to wage war.

All human beings are born with the same capacity for expressing emotions, but there is an individual variation in the intensity of the influence that each emotion has on the overall function of the mind. For example, in some people rage and anger may have a stronger influence than compassion and tolerance. Likewise, in others greed, jealousy, and selfishness may mute the influence of other advanced emotions. Therefore, the Emotional Division is the major deciding factor for the individual differences among human beings. This division is also responsible for the overall disposition, attitude, and outlook of a person. In fact, it is the Emotional Division that generates the necessary drive to initiate an action. Without emotions, human beings would remain passive reactionaries. With emotions, we are aggressive activists.

The Emotional Division of the human mind shapes our character and our response to the environment. Just imagine if human beings did not have emotions. We would be reduced to nature-created robots—expressionless, mechanical zombies programmed to survive. To illustrate, suppose a person crashes his car into a group of people, causing many injuries and deaths. Obviously, the car, being a mechanical contraption, cannot show any emotion. It is under the control of the driver and does what it is directed to do. The driver, being in possession of an emotional division, might exhibit various responses to having caused an accident, including grief, sorrow, fear, remorse, self-loathing, among others. The driver may fear for his safety, and feel that the dire consequences—physical, legal, financial—are overwhelming. The Emotional Division sets the tone and directs the Intellectual Division to come up with a plan of action. The Intellectual Division may then determine that running from the accident scene is the appropriate response. Fear, an emotion, sets the tone, but the actual flight response is concocted and implemented in the Intellectual Division. In an alternative scenario, the emotions of grief and compassion may lead the Intellectual Division to choose a different action—helping the victims and calling for an ambulance. It is the Emotional Division, not the Intellectual Division, that most sets us apart from lower animals.

The Instinctual Division

The Instinctual Division is the unconscious counterpart of the Intellectual and Emotional divisions. This division plays a crucial role in our struggle for survival as it holds the directives from nature. Nature expresses its intent through the Instinctual Division via three basic directives: (1) protection of self, (2) preservation of the surrounding environment to support the self, and (3) propagation of the self. These fundamental directives from nature are incorporated in our mind as basic instincts—thus the name Instinctual Division. However, in the case of humans, nature has expanded this division to accommodate countless useful acquired or learned habits. Here's the catch: only when the intellect and the emotions are in harmony can an individual recognize his talents and be able to polish them as tools of survival. Therefore, a pragmatic outlook and a healthy attitude are essential in the struggle for survival.

For lower animals, whose learning capacity is limited by meager intellect and a narrow range of emotions, learned behavior pales when compared to unlearned, primary instinctual behavior. Humans are the opposite. By virtue of its having a wide array of advanced emotions, sassy primitive emotions, and a powerful and versatile intellect, learned behavior not only overshadows but also modifies unlearned primary behavior. With humans, the interpretation of nature's directives and the choice of acquired habits are largely up to the individual.

The Irrational Nature of Emotional Decision Making

For all practical purposes, there is an imaginary, active, selective, and psychogenic barrier, like the Great Wall of China, separating the Intellectual Division from the Emotional Division and the Instinctual Division. This barrier acts as a screening agent for the Emotional Division. Like any effective screener, it fully understands the Emotional Division's needs, requirements, and directives. It screens all incoming messages from the Intellectual Division and lets in only those that appeal to the emotions.

This screening agent is nonexistent at birth and does not appear until sometime during early childhood. In the beginning stages, it is a nonselective, weak barrier. As a child grows, the barrier becomes stronger and more selective. By the time the child reaches the early or midteens, the agent develops into a full-fledged selective barrier. A fully matured and operational screening agent is anything but a simple, passive barrier. Its structural integrity is guarded by the Intellectual Division, and its functional integrity is controlled by the Emotional Division. The Emotional Division dictates terms to the agent that fulfill its own needs. This arrangement leaves very little room for the Intellectual Division to force its messages through to either the Emotional Division or the Instinctual Division.

When the Emotional Division is in a state of distress or turmoil, it can block messages coming from the Intellectual Division. Rational thought is inhibited by the powerful emotional drives. No wonder when you lose your cool or composure, you cannot think or act straight. Only the Intellectual Division is capable of understanding the world we live in and assessing the situations we encounter. However, because the Intellectual Division has only conditional access to the rest of the mind, it is forced to compute its response based on the input from the Emotional Division, which can be irrational.

This interplay has great relevance to productive habits, such as playing golf or performing surgery, as well as to counterproductive habits, such as compulsive gambling. When the Intellectual Division concludes, on the other hand, that continuing to smoke presents a threat to an individual's survival, it takes a Herculean effort to convince the Emotional Division to concur.

Those who have sought my help in overcoming their gambling addictions are usually disgusted with themselves. They are ashamed of their actions. They believe that their irresponsible, ill-disciplined behavior has led to their problems. Indeed, they are so filled with self-loathing that they can't believe it isn't enough to force them to stop gambling. The reason is clear to me. Their intellects are blocked from receiving these healthy messages by the intransigent Emotional Division, which compels them to continue gambling regardless of the consequences.

The Origins of the Gambling Habit

Why do habits play such a crucial role in our lives? We live in a world that does not automatically guarantee a comfortable, secure, peaceful, and happy lifestyle for all. Life is an uphill struggle. But nature has graciously bestowed upon us the necessary ammunition in our quest to adapt to the ever-changing world and meet the demands placed on us by our immediate environment. Habits are one such gift to help us meet the omnipresent challenges. In a way, habits are like a sixth sense. They play a decisive and complex role in shaping our overall behavior patterns. They become an integral part of our lifestyle and blend with our very identities.

Let's pretend for a moment that we lived in a world without habits. Although we would have the capacity to learn the mechanics of an activity, we would not be able to retain this knowledge. Learning the same tasks again and again is monotonous, time-consuming, and self-defeating. For instance, we would be forever riding bicycles with training wheels and never learn the art of balancing a bicycle. And someone daring enough to ski an expert slope may end up licking his wounds in the hospital. And golf balls would be flying in every direction, except onto the fairways and putting greens. It wouldn't be much fun to watch sports played by eternal amateurs, and we wouldn't have many ski resorts, golf and tennis clubs, or auto races. Without the advantage of habit formation, we would be severely handicapped and restricted to performing very few tasks. Without habits we probably would not have survived the Stone Age.

Habits run the spectrum from best to worst. Interestingly enough, only human beings have to sort out good from bad habits and take extra effort to keep bad ones out of reach. Unlike animals, who rely on nature to select the right habits for them, humans have to pick theirs out of many and learn each one's mechanics to adopt it. Instead of a wide, predetermined array of primary habits, nature granted us a powerful mind with unlimited imagination and the freedom to select the habits of our choice, so that we could be the masters of our own destiny. Unfortunately, such a privilege does not come without responsibilities or boundaries. We are expected to display a great deal of diligence, discipline, responsibility, and caution in our selection process. Otherwise, we may get hurt. Depending on how we handle the selection of habits, we could turn out to be our own best friend or our worst enemy. The choice is ours to make.

We accumulate thousands of habits in our lifetime. Habits are necessary to our survival; we could not function without them. Here's the big question: what force drives us to choose one habit over another? I do not think there is a simple answer. Obviously, if we were not attracted to an activity in the first place, we would never proceed through the grueling process of converting that activity into an acquired habit. To capture our attention, it must appeal to our intellect as well as our emotions.

There are three memory banks, one assigned to each division of the mind. The entire Instinctual Division acts like a giant long-term memory bank. Primary habits by definition are formed in a mysterious fashion and deposited in the Instinctual Division during the developmental stages of an organism. There is no way to figure out how, when, and where these original primary instincts formed. They come to us at birth for us to use wisely.

Acquired habits are formed in the Intellectual Division and are then transferred to the Instinctual Division as images. The memory bank of the Intellectual Division is dynamic and volatile, and experiences constant shifts. The messages in this memory bank have a short life span. Frequent reinforcement is needed to retain the messages here for longer than the usual period of time. The messages in this bank have two options. Either they are expelled completely, or they are converted into biological memory chips, screened through the Emotional Division and imprinted in the Instinctual Division. This concept is extremely important in our learning process, because emotional balance will keep the pathway open for the transportation of the memory chip from the Intellectual Division to the Instinctual Division. This is one of many reasons why people learn faster when they are emotionally stable.

Why Do Humans Develop Destructive Habits?

What distinguishes the person who throws caution and cultural standards to the wind and engages in addictive behaviors, such as reckless gambling, even when he risks ostracism and financial ruin? The personality traits and mental disposition of an addict will eventually determine the course of his bondage. Often, the initial motivation of the person is curiosity or rebellion. A young person may gamble with his friends because it's cool or gives him a thrill. But it is what happens next that determines whether he will develop a passion for gambling recklessly.

Since none of us is born with addictive habits, and they are not necessary for our survival, how do they become entrenched? Modern behavioral scientists have provided many clues to the course of addiction—such as an individual's inherent affinity for a particular habit, personality traits, socioeconomic status, educational background, and cultural views, and, finally, the nature of the addictive habit itself. Genetic factors are known to play a role in a person's affinity for a particular addictive habit.

Tendencies are not inevitabilities, however, and socioeconomic factors only go so far to explain addiction. By and large, exposure to an addictive habit ranks number one among various causative factors, but it certainly doesn't explain the mysterious origins and drives of addictive habits. Even those with all the odds against them do not necessarily become addicts. For a habit to form, the Emotional Division of the mind must first be primed to crave relief through addictive behavior. It must be provoked by an internal need, what I call an addictive drive: a sense of deprivation, entitlement, invincibility, disenchantment, insecurity, or defiance.

Animals of a lower intellectual order have been provided with the requisite primary habits for survival, but they are less capable of learning from exposure to the environment. For example, birds migrate to the south in the winter months, because they are driven by their primary habits; the polar bear knows how to handle subzero temperatures through hibernation. If human beings, on the other hand, were to rely on their basic primary habits to survive in similar temperatures, we would end up as frozen Popsicles. Nature fine-tunes the behavior of animals except human beings through their primary habits. Because animals mainly operate from primary habits, with very little modification and manipulation from the Intellectual Division, their overall behavior is predictable and consistent with species-specific responses. In contrast, human beings have to rely more on their acquired habits than their primary habits for one reason: they are bestowed with a powerful intellect, a vivid imagination, and unlimited freedom to choose their way of life.

But the freedom that we enjoy does not come cheap. Nature has warned us that we are accountable for our actions and will be punished if we misbehave. Furthermore, nature controls the type of punitive action and time frame for dispensing consequences. For example, everyone knows that we pay a heavy price for selecting bad habits such as reckless gambling. Bad habits can inflict irrevocable damage on a person and bring misery not only to the individual involved but also to others in close association with that person. Unfortunately, nature refuses to listen to our explanations and excuses for selecting bad habits. Without exceptions, nature dispenses appropriate penalties for our misdeeds. We must endure the consequences of our own bad choices.

Most important, remember that once a habit is established, it is impossible to erase the image from the mind. At best we can tame the influence of an unwanted habit. A person has to expend a lot of energy, effort, and time to manifest a small victory over an entrenched, unwanted bad habit. Because we rely on our acquired habits for survival, what we learn has a major impact on our behavior and existence.

Based on my observation of different characteristics of all addictive habits, I have classified them into three primary categories:

1. Mind-soothing addictive habits
2. Mind-altering addictive habits
3. Mind-provoking addictive habits

MIND-SOOTHING ADDICTIVE HABITS

Cigarette smoking, drinking coffee or tea, compulsive eating, and sex fall into this category. The comforting and soothing effects of these activities captivate the attention of an individual and tie him or her to these habits. The unique feature of these habits is that they allow the mental status to remain intact. For instance, a cigarette smoker does not lose mental balance like an alcoholic. The dangers that accompany these habits are well hidden, and thus they appear harmless. It is not easy for the individual to identify and acknowledge the harmful effects of these habits even after years of associating with them. By providing a false sense of security, these habits con the individual into remaining loyal for years.

For instance, even after decades of aggressive campaigns against the smoking habit because of the related health hazards, millions of people all over the world still smoke without any reservation. Similarly, despite all the research on health problems related to obesity, Americans are getting fatter by the day, and billions of dollars are being spent on treating obesity. The ever-increasing number of teenage pregnancies, sexually transmitted diseases, and sex-related immoral and illegal acts also exemplify the hidden, long-term costs of mind-soothing addictions.

MIND-ALTERING ADDICTIVE HABITS

Some of the most notorious, mind-crippling, and unhealthy habits belong to this group. They include alcohol and various drugs. All of these habits are based on chemical substance abuse of one type or another. Besides providing the expected comfort, euphoria, ecstasy, and thrill, the addictive chemical substances affect and alter the mental status to a lesser or greater degree. People who are involved with these habits experience temporary or permanent impairment of memory, mental balance, reasoning, judgment, and physical reflexes. These habits adversely affect an individual physically, mentally, and spiritually. Eventually, addicts may end up as mental cripples and physical invalids. The substances that are incriminated with these habits range from so-called soft drugs, such as alcohol, Valium, codeine, barbiturates, and marijuana, to hard drugs such as cocaine, crack, heroin, PCP, and methamphetamines.

MIND-PROVOKING ADDICTIVE HABITS

There are certain issues about a human being that one can spend centuries trying to explain in logical terms, but they will still remain a mystery. Mind-provoking addictive habits are one such entity. The striking feature of these addictions is that there are no visible and physical mediating agents such as alcohol, cigarettes, food, or sex to evoke an addictive response.

There is no tangible explanation for the power of these habits. Rather, people are hooked on an "idea." For example, some people are hooked on the idea of basking in unlimited wealth and power, which is the basis of this type of addiction. The persistent idea keeps these addicts running in circles because their target is an unreachable goal. Not realizing this fact, they embark on a never-ending journey into oblivion. The insatiable desire to reach their goal at any cost provokes these addicts to concoct extraordinary measures and to implement them without fail. The actions they undertake without knowing what the outcome could be gives these people a greater thrill than reaching their destination. The euphoria and the thrill couched in the action they take keep them going forever, and, believe it or not, these addicts cannot get off this roller coaster ride.

A compulsive gambler cannot stop gambling even if he is on a winning streak, since his expectations are limitless. If he loses, he continues to play to make up for his losses. Win or lose, the mind-provoking addiction will not give an individual the needed gratification and satisfaction to release him from its stranglehold. Despite the absence of physical mediating agents, these addictions are extremely powerful and will not let a person go without sapping his spirits, hopes, and future. Eventually, he ends up restless, agitated, sleepless, and preoccupied with his addiction just as a cocaine, crack, or heroin addict would be.

The Drive to Gamble

To be effective against the gambling habit, we must focus on the invisible enemy—the internally generated drives that feed the habit. By focusing on the external features, a gambler may stop the activity for a time but will never get rid of the compulsion or the desire to gamble. As long as the compulsion is alive, he will eventually return to the habit. You cannot get rid of a habit by simply getting rid of the offending activity.

The key to unproductive habits such as compulsive gambling is identified in six Addictive Profiles (see Step 3), which are actually persuasive stories people tell themselves to justify unproductive behaviors. The emotional drive of these stories allows them to continue behaviors that the rational mind clearly acknowledges as destructive. These drives are all-consuming. Often a person will have more than one. They trigger the Emotional Division to seek relief. They include:

- **The Deprivation Drive:** A persistent emptiness and the intense need for a pacifier to give comfort and security.
- **The Entitlement Drive:** The belief that one deserves to "let go," release stress, and pursue excitement, even when the behavior is destructive to self and others.
- **The Invincibility Drive:** The illusion that one will be spared the consequences of the addictive behavior and will ultimately triumph in spite of it.
- **The Disenchantment Drive:** The deep disappointment in a world that does not meet one's expectations, which drives one to seek escape from reality.

- **The Insecurity Drive:** An overwhelming fear and sense of inadequacy that require constant bolstering.
- **The Defiance Drive:** A deep-seated gesture of rebelliousness that persists in behavior long after the need for rebellion has passed.

One or more of these drives fuels the gambling habit. Even if the compulsive gambler is prevented from gambling, the addiction will remain as long as the addictive drives are present. The nucleus persists—the overwhelming sense of deprivation, entitlement, invincibility, disenchantment, insecurity, and defiance that gave rise to the addiction in the first place. The same dynamic holds true with all bad habits. They are invariably the result of self-stories created by the mind.

The Emotional Division plays tricks on compulsive gamblers to the extent that they rarely understand where the drive to gamble is coming from. John, a thirty-two-year-old freelance electrician, who sought my help with his gambling problem, was such a person. John was a single man who lived alone. He'd had many girlfriends, but his relationships were always short-term. He said that he intended to marry and have a family someday, if he found the right girl. For me, that was an immediate red flag. Whenever a person says, at thirty-two, that he is still on the lookout for the right mate, the alarm goes off in my head. I ask myself, Why has this person been unable to find a partner? Are his standards too high? Is he too picky? Is he unwilling to compromise? Does he distrust people? Is he looking in all the wrong places?

I focused my interview with John on this issue, because I believed it would shed some light on his priorities, expectations, outlook, and attitude. In fact, his problem with relationships was directly related to his compulsive gambling problem.

John was reasonably happy and comfortable with his profession. He was free from other addictive habits. He'd tried cocaine, pot, and alcohol in his teens but had never got hooked on any of them. He was not taking any prescription medications. His main problem was that he could not stop betting on horse races. He said, "I am self-employed and have my own schedule, but if I don't make my deadlines and make my customers happy, I will be out of business. Lately, my pull toward the horse races is distracting me from my work, and I cannot afford to be preoccupied, especially when I am dealing with electrical power lines. If I don't straighten up my act, you may hear in the news one day that an electrician died on the job through electrocution. In a sense, I am committing myself to the electric chair. Please, Dr. Prasad, spare me from being electrocuted."

I sat back for a few seconds, thinking. What was wrong with this picture? John seemed to be a levelheaded, hardworking, sensible individual. What was going on? I asked him to tell me about his childhood.

John grew up as one of four children, but he was always something of a loner. When he was young, the family lived in upstate New York, close to a horse farm. He fell in love with the horses, and he told me he'd loved them more than any of the people in his life. "You can trust animals but not people," he said. "Animals will never deceive you."

When John was seventeen, he fell in love with a girl. She liked him but was not in love with him. They went out for a few months, and one day she dumped him for another guy. He was deeply hurt by this incident and, gradually, he shifted his time and energy to the horses. The farm's owner liked John, and he let him ride in exchange for helping around the farm. Occasionally, a horse would be sold for racing, but John wasn't that interested in the sport. In fact, he was twenty-five before he saw his first race.

One day, he and a girl he was dating decided to go to the races. John made a point of going to the stables to take a look at the horses beforehand. One horse captured his attention, and he bet on that horse, even though it had a lousy track record. "Don't worry," he told his date. "He won't let me down." His horse finished in the middle, and John lost a few dollars. But instead of being turned off, he got emotionally attached to the horse. At that moment he established a pattern for betting with his heart, not with his head. Over the years, he repeated the process over and over. He won a few times, but he lost more often. John never lost much money. He wasn't ever in debt. But the emotional pull toward the horses distracted him more than the money involved. Sometimes John would get attached to a particular horse and follow it to different racetracks around the country. Even if the horse lost, he would visit the horse and tell him that he still believed in him.

John recognized that his behavior was not normal, but he said he got a strong thrill from watching his favorite horse run. All of his emotional energy was tied up in the horse. He had no other real social life. He knew something had to be done.

I knew it would not be easy for me to help John switch his attention from animals to his fellow human beings. I had to guide him to be more sensible and pragmatic, and less sensitive and sentimental.

"There is no guarantee that you won't be betrayed in your relationships," I told him, "but you have to take calculated chances in life. That's what human interaction is all about. You think you can avoid hurt and protect yourself by shutting people out, but it won't work."

I explained to John that his habit of getting carried away emotionally went beyond horses. He would have to work on that tendency if he wanted a normal relationship with his fellow human beings. "Betting on a horse can be entertaining, but for you it is exhausting, stressful, and destructive. You've invested too much of yourself emotionally."

John shook his head slowly. "Dr. Prasad, I'm not stupid," he said. "So how come I would bet on a losing horse again and again?"

"Well," I told him, "I think it worked something like this. When you were emotionally attached to a horse, and could not bear the thought of the horse losing, you would increase your bet in the belief that you were empowering that horse. Unfortunately, a horse cannot pick up speed just because someone in the gallery is rooting for it. Horses, like humans, have limitations. No matter how hard you cheer, the horse can only do its best, and sometimes that's not good enough."

Something in my words broke through to John, because he started laughing. "I can't believe myself," he said. "What was I thinking?"

"You were thinking with your heart," I replied. "And that's trouble."

I worked with John, using the six steps outlined in this book. When we finished our work together, he remained determined to pursue a healthy, meaningful life.

Two years later, I got a call from John saying that he had stopped betting on horses altogether and had no intention of betting again. For the last six months he'd been dating a young woman who was a registered nurse. He sounded quite content.

◇◈◇◈◇◈◇◈◇◈◇◈◇◈◇◈◇◈◇◈◇◈◇◈◇◈◇◈

The Two Faces
of Reckless Gambling

ALL RECKLESS GAMBLERS fall into two major groups: *compulsive*, reckless gamblers and *noncompulsive*, reckless gamblers. Compulsive, reckless gamblers are driven by the idea of *making* money. Noncompulsive, reckless gamblers are driven by the idea of *spending* money. The chart on the following page outlines the differences between the two types of reckless gamblers: compulsive and noncompulsive.

The Compulsive, Reckless Gambler:
A Drive to Win

Compulsive gamblers operate outside the realm of reality and are not in touch with the consequences of their actions. Some experts believe that compulsive gamblers really want to lose—that deep down they are trying to punish themselves. I do not

COMPULSIVE, RECKLESS GAMBLERS	NONCOMPULSIVE, RECKLESS GAMBLERS
1. Even though they envision a lavish lifestyle, their obsession is on making money.	1. They have a penchant for spending beyond their means, thus compromising their security.
2. They direct their own personal and borrowed resources, primarily to bring in more money.	2. To support spending habits, they borrow recklessly rather than paying more attention to earning money.
3. They get immense thrill and elation from the actions of betting on volatile ventures.	3. They get a good deal of pleasure from spending lavishly, without paying any attention to the consequences of their actions.
4. Besides the action, even the uncertainty of the end result gives them a tremendous thrill. The greater the uncertainty, the more excited they become.	4. They do not get any kind of pleasure from actions directed at generating funds to support their spending habit.
5. They believe they are invincible and will ultimately win big.	5. They feel entitled to have more, and justify their wild spending by the belief that they deserve it.
6. They feel a strong sense of deprivation when they are not playing games of chance.	6. They are disenchanted by life as they find it.
7. Invariably, they have more than one addictive habit—such as alcohol or drugs as well.	7. Usually, they do not show any signs of addiction to substances like cocaine, alcohol, heroin, pot, amphetamines, etc. There may be an addiction, if any, to smoking cigarettes.
8. They are more likely to have a criminal record.	8. They usually do not have criminal records.
9. Because of their basic personality traits, and the presence of other addictive habits, it is much harder to help them overcome their addictions.	9. It is relatively easy to help these individuals to alter their behavior for the better.

COMPULSIVE, RECKLESS GAMBLERS	NONCOMPULSIVE, RECKLESS GAMBLERS
10. There is a strong psychological withdrawal symptom, as well as variable degrees of physical withdrawals, depending on associated addictions. This makes it harder for them during the first few days of change. 11. Recurrence rate of original behavior is around 40–50 percent, even after one year.	10. There are very few physical and psychological withdrawal symptoms during the initial stages of change. 11. Recurrence rate of original behavior is around 10–20 percent, provided an individual has turned around his life for the better and remains stable for at least one year.

buy this argument. In my practice, even the most compulsive, reckless gamblers, who have lost everything in life, admit that they gamble to win, not lose. The focus is on the activity itself, not on the end result. Without hesitation, every one of them concurs that the gambling action is important. The few moments of uncertainty boost adrenaline levels, and they all literally experience a rush similar to a shot of heroin for a drug addict. Compulsive, reckless gamblers get an almost ejaculatory thrill from the activity of gambling, and possess a bold confidence that one day, sooner or later, they will hit the big jackpot. Because of the thrill of the action, and the strong belief that they will hit it big one day, these individuals are not willing to get off the roller-coaster ride once they get on. Literally, the action sequence and anticipation of a definite positive result possess the mind of reckless gamblers and drive them to become addicted to the cycle of events. That is the reason why, win or lose, they cannot stop gambling. The thrill grows as the stakes get higher.

Is compulsive gambling a kind of sickness? I believe that it is an extreme form of psychological aberration, not a mental sickness. Do compulsive gamblers experience withdrawal symptoms like other hard-core addicts, when they are deprived of the activity? Yes, they do. Abstention from gambling triggers a strong psychological withdrawal syndrome. These individuals get agitated, upset, annoyed, restless, and sleep-deprived if they refrain from gambling for extended periods.

Even the uncertainty about the future, which each of us is supposed to take in good stride, excites the compulsive reckless gambler. The higher the level of uncertainty, the greater the thrill. Most of us have learned to balance our desires for security and excitement. For example, if you invest in a steady, income-producing municipal bond, there is more security but less thrill. On the other hand, if you invest in high-yield volatile bonds or stocks, there is more thrill but less security. A responsible gambler would lean toward safety first, thrill later. I believe that for a compulsive reckless gambler, the emphasis is on the thrill and uncertainty, not the security.

It is hard for most people to imagine that playing a simple game of odds can wreck a person's life. Just like hard-core drug addicts, many compulsive gamblers have lost their jobs, families, and entire life savings to their habit. Most of the time, compulsive gamblers are overconfident that their future will not be affected by their compulsion. They are in a state of denial.

I have treated many compulsive, reckless gamblers. Although they share behaviors in common, there is a tremendous variation in their reasons for gambling and the paths they travel to reach their unhappy destinations. One thing is for sure: when people behave irrationally, they have their own reasons for their behavior, even when these reasons don't make sense. To be successful, I must reach deep into their minds and discover those reasons.

Charles, a forty-five-year-old stockbroker-turned-investment banker, was typical of many of the compulsive gamblers I've treated over the years. He started out as a responsible gambler, briefly passed through a period of recreational gambling, and finally ended up as a compulsive reckless gambler. When he came to see me, he said that because of his compulsive gambling binges in Las Vegas and Atlantic City, he had lost his business edge. Charles managed a large mutual fund, but for the past three years the value of his mutual fund had taken a downturn. The more perturbed he became about his business, the stronger the pull he felt to escape the harsh reality by frequenting casinos. Charles had been miscalculating the direction of the financial institutions that he was investing in, and his calls were off the mark. He knew he was losing his grip. He wanted to get his act together before it was too late. Besides, he already knew he would have to crawl back on his hands and knees to take charge of his life once again. He was willing to do this, but he needed guidance.

Charles was one of four children. His father was a successful financial manager. His parents had divorced when he was fourteen. He and two other siblings stayed with his mother, and his older brother stayed with his father.

After Charles graduated with a degree in finance and marketing, his father offered him a job at his firm. Charles hesitated. He'd never liked his father, whom he'd found to be a cold, demanding control freak. But the money was great, so, against his better judgment, he accepted his father's offer.

Charles joined the business with lots of enthusiasm, but no matter how well he performed, instead of offering encouragement his father criticized and humiliated him. "My father systematically stripped me of my dignity, honor, and confidence," he said. "After three years, I could not tolerate his mental abuse, so I moved out on my own. It took me one year just to regain my confidence. Luckily, I had developed a wonderful networking system. It wasn't hard to find people who disliked my father and were more than willing to help me start my own business. It was tough in the beginning, but within four years I was doing very well. My mutual fund took off like a rocket. Sometimes I worked sixteen hours a day."

I observed that Charles was ambitious, goal-oriented, hardworking, and well organized. "I see you have inherited many of your father's qualities," I told him with a smile.

Charles didn't like to hear that, but it was true. In a strange way he was a close replica of his father. The only difference between them, as I saw it, was that his father was very cold and lacking in compassion, whereas Charles was more sentimental and sensitive. The harsh working environment and the shallow narcissistic people in the business world did not bother his father, but the same environment did affect Charles. Even though his business was fine and he had a good marriage, inside he was emotionally uncomfortable. This discomfort got him into trouble.

One day, in a casual conversation with one of his country club friends, Charles mentioned that he was exhausted and needed a break. His friend invited him to join him on a weekend excursion to Las Vegas. Charles accepted, and they spent three days wining and dining, seeing shows, and playing a few hands of poker and blackjack.

Charles had a wonderful time. It was totally relaxing, and because he was a very careful and smart player, he won $3,000 at the tables. In the end he boasted to his friend that it wasn't a bad deal. Not only had he had a good time, he'd made a profit! Charles hadn't known that making money could be so much fun—and that was the initial hook. From that day on, he was a frequent visitor to the casinos.

In the beginning, Charles would spend some time relaxing over dinner and enjoying a show before he hit the tables. But as time passed, he was more interested in playing card games and less interested in the entertainment and relaxation. Once he switched priorities, he started to lose money. The more he lost, the more aggressive his bets became.

"Nowadays," he said, "I bet on these games like a crazy person. The more I bet, the more I lose. The more I lose, the more I bet. Every time I lose, I'm distraught for a few seconds. But then I'm eager to bet more to recover my losses. I don't seem to be able to pull out of this compulsive, vicious cycle. I need your help before it is too late."

I considered Charles's situation. Would I be able to devise a rescue plan? After several days, I decided I could help Charles, for several reasons:

First, I observed that Charles was a proud, stubborn, and intelligent man. Pride and stubbornness are like double-edged swords. They can be useful tools for survival, or sharp weapons of self-destruction. He was using them as weapons for self-destruction, but I thought he would be open to turning them around to his benefit.

Second, Charles was smart enough to recognize he was on his way to losing everything that he had built over the last twenty years. He hadn't yet hit bottom, and he wanted to get out of the hole before this happened. He was willing to work hard and go through whatever hardships were necessary to save himself from total annihilation. He wanted to prove to himself that he could turn back.

Third, even though Charles drank wine occasionally, he had never lost control over his alcohol consumption. If he had been addicted to any mind-altering substances, such as cocaine or alcohol, it would have been harder to help him.

Fourth, his marriage was still intact. Charles and his wife had a strained relationship after years of Charles's neglect, but they were still functioning as a family, and Charles was willing to do what it took to repair the damage.

The big question was, How did a savvy, hardworking guy like Charles lose his bearing in the first place? I felt the answer was tied to his tumultuous relationship with his father. He admired his father's professional prowess, but despised his disposition and character. It was a love-hate relationship—he loved to hate his father. These strong emotions began to shape his behavior. An extreme degree of love or hatred locks an individual into the orbit of the other person. Charles's underlying animosity for his father began when his parents divorced, and it became a full-fledged hatred when he went to work for him.

During the three years Charles worked for his father, he was chastised and ridiculed. The two words his father used—"numskull" and "loser"—were etched in his mind. Probably, he was driven to professional success more by his hatred toward his father than his love of the profession. He wanted to prove to his father that he was not a numskull or a loser. But no matter how successful Charles was, it was never enough. His father's words never stopped ringing in his head. In fact, his strong negative emotions exhausted him more than his workload.

The first time Charles won in Las Vegas, it set the stage for his future compulsion to go back there again. He was in the art of making money. So why not make money while you are relaxing. However, by the third or fourth time, his stream of luck headed southward. Like all compulsive gamblers, he convinced himself that his luck would change. But once his losses started to pile up to the $10,000 to $15,000 mark, he became serious. Now he was bent on recovering the lost money. The deeper his losses, the more desperate he became. At that point it was not about the loss of money, but about his father's voice in his head, saying, "You're a numskull and a loser," if he stopped gambling after a $15,000 loss.

In the end, with his losses piling up, he truly felt in his mind that his father was probably right. He was a numskull and a loser. His spirit was completely deflated.

To get out of this destructive cycle, Charles would have to free himself from his father's hold. It wasn't enough for him to force himself to stop his destructive behavior. He had to slay the demons that drove him to gamble in the first place. By rigorous adherence to my method, he was able to do this.

Anyone can become a reckless, compulsive gambler, but the truth of the matter is that this addiction most commonly afflicts people who are down on their luck, drifting through life, and unable to cope with the stresses and hardships that come their way.

Tom, a thirty-seven-year-old merchant marine, fit into this category. When Tom came to see me, his addiction to gambling was hurting him in many ways. First, he had accumulated approximately $30,000 in gambling debts. Second, his wife was threatening to divorce him. Third, people who owned his debts were threatening to hurt him or his family. Fourth, he was making a lot of mistakes at work because he was distraught, and he would lose his job if he continued down this path. Fifth, his behavior was affecting his personal health in the form of stomach ulcers. Sixth, like pouring fuel over fire, he had started to drink more alcohol than ever to drown his troubles. Lately, he had even been drinking on the job.

A few months before he came to see me, Tom had sought help from Gamblers Anonymous. He was a proud man and he did not like to tell other people his pathetic life story. So he stopped going to those meetings. He said he was desperate and begged me to take him as a patient.

I encouraged Tom to tell me about himself. He was a high school graduate, married for ten years, and the father of two girls, ages seven and five. He had worked for the merchant marines for the last twelve years. Before he joined the merchant marines, he had worked odd jobs in the construction industry. He told me he was a good handyman and liked carpentry, but a downturn in the economy had forced him to look for other work. He'd joined the merchant marines because the pay and benefits were extremely good. The only problem was that he had to be away from home for a couple of months at a stretch. Between trips, he would spend three to five weeks at home.

In the beginning, Tom found the job exciting because he had the opportunity to visit many countries. But after a few years, the thrill of traveling had worn off and was replaced by boredom. The weeks spent on the high seas were getting on his nerves. At times, he felt this was not the life he had dreamed about. He wanted to change his job, but could not find a suitable one that would pay the same amount he was making. He and his family were accustomed to the comforts that his salary afforded. It was difficult for them to adjust to lower standards.

One day, while at sea, one of Tom's friends talked him into betting on an ongoing basketball game to have some fun. The idea appealed to him because, throughout his life, he had been an ardent basketball fan. As a child he had often gone to games with his father. Many times he'd noticed his father betting on games through an agent. For him, going to these games and then to a restaurant with his father and his father's friends was a pleasant ritual and a happy memory. He didn't see any harm in doing a little betting, just as his father had done.

Tom recalled that day on the ship clearly, because even though it was a small wager, he was on the edge of his seat until the game was over. Those few hours were exciting to him. When his team was behind, he began to cheer for them to win. He had no recollection of the end result of the game, but he remembered the thrill. In due course, Tom and his shipmates started to bet on basketball games on a regular basis. In the off-season, they would bet on other sports. Besides betting on these games with his shipmates, Tom also started to bet with a professional agent. Small wagers slowly turned into larger bets. As soon as the ship came ashore, his agents would be waiting to collect on his debts. He would go to the bank, cash his paycheck, and either pay off the full amount or a partial amount with a promise to pay the remainder at a later date. That is how his gambling debts started to pile up. Like many compulsive gamblers, Tom would experience the rush when he bet on a game. The more money he put down, the greater the rush. He started to raise the stakes. He won a few wagers, but more often he lost. As the years passed, Tom began to take home less and less money. When his wife, Emily, questioned his diminishing paycheck, he lied and said that the shipping company was in financial trouble and all the employees had taken a pay cut. He promised her that it was only temporary. Emily believed him, and she took a part-time job to make up the difference.

Tom felt terrible about his lie, and he was disgusted with himself for his weakness. He decided to stop betting. For the next four weeks, while he was on the ship, he managed to refrain. But to his surprise, he began to experience an overwhelming psychological withdrawal. He was agitated and grouchy, and could not focus on his work or sleep well. He also felt frightened about his huge debt and didn't know how he would pay it. To forget his plight, Tom began to drink heavily.

One day, while he was drunk, he called his agent and bet on a game. The cycle started all over again. In the midst of his betting frenzy, he observed an interesting change in himself. Since he had begun betting heavily, he had lost all desire to go to basketball games. Many times when he was ashore, he had an opportunity to go, but decided to stay home instead. In fact, his wife used to joke about his love for the game, saying if he had a choice between making love to her or going to a game, he would pick the latter. Sitting in my office, defeated and sad, Tom said those days had become a distant memory, and he wished he could relive them once again. He felt it was possible with my help.

I thought about what Tom had told me. Deep down, I was not convinced that he had the wherewithal to turn his life around. Besides, he was drinking a lot of liquor. Even though he was not an overt alcoholic, his level of consumption would hinder any chances of recovery. Considering these points, I felt it would take an enormous amount of energy, conviction, and discipline to pull out of the deep hole he had dug for himself.

I believe in being honest, up-front, and blunt with my patients. I told Tom that if I accepted him as my patient, I might be wasting his time and money. Even with my help, his chances for recovery were slim. But he insisted that I take him as my patient. He said that he'd tried everything and that I was his last hope.

After a few seconds of silence, I challenged Tom to give me one good reason why I should take him as my patient. He looked straight into my eyes and said, "You asked for one and I'll give you two." Then he stood up and hurried out of my office. This happened in a split second, and I didn't know what was going on. But it became clear to me when Tom promptly returned with his two daughters. He said, "Dr. Prasad, aren't these two good enough reasons? For their sake, I must clean up my act. Every time I bet on a game, I am robbing them of a good future. I make a lot of money, and if I stop gambling, I can save for their college education and give them an opportunity for a good life."

I was moved by Tom's words and convinced of his sincerity. Although I knew that it would be an uphill battle, Tom would have a fighting chance because his passion for his daughters' future was stronger than his passion for gambling.

In the coming months, I saw Tom on several occasions. He was seriously executing the plan I gave him, and his spirits were buoyed by the results. He also said that he and his wife were a lot closer than ever before. He was admiring and appreciating his wife for her patience and courage. He was also gratified that his friends were so happy to see him after his long absence. They told him that the construction industry was booming. One of his friends was thinking of opening up his own company in the next couple of years, and he suggested that Tom might join him as a partner.

Meanwhile, Tom took a job onshore for a cut in pay, and he moonlighted on some evenings and weekends doing carpentry on construction projects. By the six-month mark, he was doing very well.

I didn't hear from Tom for six years; then one day I had a phone message that his wife had called. I returned the call with some trepidation. I wondered if Tom had started betting again, and if his wife was calling for help. I was pleasantly surprised when she stated the reason for her call. "I wanted to thank you, Dr. Prasad. You saved our family. Tom paid off his last gambling debt yesterday, and our lives have never been better."

THE CHILD GAMBLER: AN ADDICT IN THE MAKING?

If playing poker or betting on horses occasionally is acceptable, at what age is it appropriate for someone to start participating in these activities? I cannot give you a specific numerical figure. It is an individual's mental state and financial state that are the deciding factors. If an individual is reasonably emotionally mature and pays his own way, he can probably gamble safely and responsibly. If a person is not self-supporting, he shouldn't be engaging in these activities.

In American society, however, there is an alarming trend involving kids in junior high and high school playing poker for recreation. Too often these students are in the habit of drinking alcohol during the games. Alcohol and poker are a deadly combination for kids.

Young boys are especially vulnerable because the poker game is glamorized on ESPN and the Internet. Remember how, fifty years ago, famous actors and actresses posed for pictures with cigarettes? The glamorization of smoking encouraged young people to pick up the habit. The same phenomenon is repeating itself in the form of gambling. The impressionable youths see big-timers with their dark glasses and million-dollar piles of chips playing poker on ESPN, and they want to imitate them. Since our society has no objection to publicly airing events like *World Poker* and *Celebrity Poker* on TV, we should not be surprised at the increase in the number of young poker players. But what surprises me most is the lack of concern voiced by parents and experts in human behavior, who insist that they see no harm in young people taking part in these games, as long as the stakes are modest. I once heard a mother state that she approved of her junior-high-school son playing poker because she thought the game would sharpen his mathematical and concentration skills. Talk about denial! The ignorance of this viewpoint is hard to fathom.

It is too early to say how many of these teenage poker players will end up as compulsive reckless gamblers—although current statistics show teenage compulsive gamblers account for about 12 percent of the total. One thing is certain: these kids do not understand their boundaries or the full consequences of their actions. Their emotions are still raw and developing, and the surrounding environment can have a great impact on their future behavior.

Many experts believe that compulsive gambling usually begins during the adolescence period and develops into a full-fledged habit in due course. It is predominantly a male habit, and the tendency to gamble on a compulsive basis runs very deep. One of my patients, whom I treated for gambling, concurred that he started to gamble on sports events at the age of ten. Craig recognized the thrill of gambling almost immediately. He was full of bravado and believed that he had an uncanny talent for picking winners. He felt that gambling gave him a chance to enhance his image by spending lavishly on his friends with his winnings.

(continued)

Craig had an underlying feeling of insecurity and an inflated sense of self-worth. He also craved recognition. He essentially bribed his friends to like him, but his efforts were futile because he could never see himself as inherently lovable.

Chasing his illusion was gratifying at first, but eventually Craig lost his way. His friends moved on, but he remained stuck in his habit. Through hard work, and with the help of my treatments, he began to improve, but it was a slow and tedious process. Despite his conscious desire to change for the better, Craig found that his mind—especially his Emotional Division— resisted change at every step of the way.

Most of my patients tell me they first got hooked on their habits—be they drinking, smoking, drugs, or gambling—in their teenage years. The kids always started innocently enough but soon they found the appeal of the activities great and eventually came to rely on them for comfort or thrills.

Playing poker at a young and immature age is especially destructive because it fosters an aggressive, cocky, self-centered, and brash mentality. There is a good chance that a youngster's future behavior will be strongly influenced by these personality traits.

My advice to parents is to let their children play more benign card games such as gin rummy or crazy eights. As a general rule, any card game played in the casinos should not be introduced to children. To spice up the benign card games, however, one can introduce reasonable noncash incentives to improve the kids' mathematical and logic skills, and to teach sportsmanship.

The Noncompulsive, Reckless Gambler: A Drive to Spend

One does not have to be a regular patron of casinos, OTB, or racetracks to be a reckless gambler. Any individual who acts first and thinks later, or doesn't even think about the consequences of his actions, is a reckless gambler.

I recently read an article in *The New York Times* about members of the armed forces and their escapades with high interest, cash-in-advance payroll loans. The article focused on the plight of a young navy petty officer and her husband from Puget Sound naval base near Seattle, Washington. This couple landed in a big mess when they fell victim to easy-access loans from quick loan outlets around the base. In fact, there are hundreds of these outlets surrounding military bases all over the country.

This couple, like many of their friends, started their careers in the navy, earning a biweekly, fixed salary. After taxes, their pay did not stretch very far. They were barely able to make ends meet.

During the summer, they were planning a visit from relatives, and they didn't have any money to entertain them. Their income was too low to borrow from legitimate sources, so, without thinking of the consequences, they borrowed $500 against their next paycheck at a 390 percent annual interest rate from one of the easy-access loan outlets. They had a good time with their visitors, but the following month when they received their paycheck, it was $575 shy. Already, the cost of their $500 loan had increased by $75! As their debt grew, they began to borrow more money to cover their expenses. This is how the perpetual cycle of borrowing and spending starts, and it gains momentum as time passes. Within a few months, they had borrowed $4,000 at very high interest rates. An accountant calculated that by October, the annual interest rate for the $4,000 that they borrowed would reach an exorbitant 650 percent. By the end of October, the petty officer was about to be shipped to the Persian Gulf when she learned that they were about to lose their home to foreclosure.

The story created a big buzz in the press among those who said it was outrageous that these loan outlets preyed upon vulnerable military personnel. It was estimated that up to 26 percent of military households were trapped in a vicious spiral of borrowing at exorbitant interest rates, leading to financial and even career ruin.

Do I sympathize with them? No, I do not. These are intelligent, free adults, who chose reckless borrowing and spending because they wanted something they could not afford.

I equate reckless borrowing and spending with reckless gambling. Do I oppose lending and borrowing altogether? Of course not—I borrowed money from a bank at an affordable interest rate to buy my house, and I consider it a wise investment. It has since tripled in value. I didn't borrow money to impress my friends, to have a fancier lifestyle than I could afford, or to purchase luxuries beyond my means.

The navy couple, and many more like them, wanted instant money, but they ignored the consequences. Their behavior is similar to that of millions of people who collect credit cards like crazy and use them with abandon. The average American consumer holds at least ten credit cards, with annual interest rates between 18 and 26 percent. Credit card companies frequently target college students, offering them large lines of credit even though they have no visible income. For many of these youngsters, living a lavish life on borrowed money is an attractive proposition, like smoking or drinking alcohol. Spending beyond their means becomes a form of addictive behavior that can exact a heavy toll.

Older charge-card addicts are more inclined to be exhibiting the Disenchantment Drive, and to some extent the Entitlement Drive. Most of the people I have treated are single or divorced working women in their thirties and forties. They tend to be restless, bored, and unhappy. They dwell on their unfulfilled dreams and feel that they deserve some excitement in their lives.

Amy, a forty-four-year-old postal worker, was a case in point. Amy had been married and divorced twice, and had no children. She was depressed and often achingly lonely. She began to go to the malls just to be around other people, and found that the act of shopping made her feel like less of an outcast. Her shopping sprees started out small, but before she knew it, Amy was spending large amounts of money every week. She was buying for the sake of buying. Many of the items were useless. She told me, "Most of the time, I don't even open the packages when I get home. I just throw them into a closet." Sobbing in my office, Amy cried that she was desperate to stop her shopping sprees, but she couldn't do it alone.

By the time she came to me, Amy was deep in debt. Although she made a good salary, her credit card bills had overwhelmed her income. She owed almost $20,000 on ten cards, and the interest kept piling up. The calls from collection agencies were constant and humiliating. "Those companies are inhumane," she said angrily. "I'm trying my best to pay my debts, but they keep calling and berating me. They have no compassion."

In her mind, Amy had transferred the blame to the collection agencies. By focusing on their harsh tactics, she could feel like a victim, even though it was her irresponsibility that got her into this mess in the first place. Patients like Amy are extremely hard to treat, because they require a complete change of mentality.

"Amy," I told her sternly, "you think life has given you a special pass. Only you can float above reality, spending as much as you want without consequences. How dare those lenders ask for payment!"

She blushed at hearing the edge in my voice. "I get your point," she said, "but what do I do?"

"Stop spending money you don't have, and pay your bills," I replied. "Keep both feet firmly on the ground and embrace the

ARE YOU A RECKLESS SPENDER?

1. Do you tend to shop and spend large amounts of money during times of depression or emotional distress?
2. Do you buy excessive numbers of items that never get used, or that you already own in sufficient quantities—like clothing or household items?
3. Do you later dispose of items you purchase, even throwing them away without opening the packages?
4. Do you lie to partners, spouses, friends, and family about your shopping and the amount of money you spent?
5. Do you run up large debts or buy unnecessary items instead of paying your bills?
6. Do you borrow or steal money to shop?
7. Do you acquire as many credit cards as you can and use them until you've reached the limit?
8. Is your shopping or spending habit interfering with work or relationships?

harsh realities of life. If you do, your spirits can never be dampened, and you don't have to resort to going on spending sprees to feel good."

THE RECKLESS BORROWING DISORDER

Reckless borrowing is a variation on reckless spending. Borrowing is fundamental to human existence because no individual is in possession of all he needs for survival. The ancient system of bartering evolved from the need to share goods and services. But what if someone had no resources to barter? The system of borrowing and lending emerged as a solution to this problem, and over the eons it has become a dizzyingly complex system. Today, it involves millions of people and trillions of dollars in an elaborate dance of debt. Foremost in this system is the invention of "plastic money," or the credit card.

Credit cards are wonderful conveniences, but they tempt human weakness. Even normally cautious, responsible spenders can get carried away with the notion that plastic money is not "real," and momentarily forget the consequences until the bill comes. They lapse into the magical thinking of a child. I remember an incident when our daughter was six. My wife and I were in a department store, discussing the pros and cons of purchasing stereo equipment. We were reluctantly concluding it was too expensive, when our daughter piped up. "If you don't have money, use your credit card," she advised. We laughed at her naïveté, but it's not so funny when rational adults subscribe to the same belief.

Credit card issuers make their profits from enormous interest rates, so they prefer customers who like to splurge. Increasingly, young adults are barraged with credit card offers. Receiving that first credit card is a memorable day in a young person's life. There is an illusion of wealth. Suddenly, they don't have to scrape and save for everything they want. The bubble may burst with the first credit card bill, or it may take longer and involve thousands of dollars in interest payments and harassing phone calls from collection agencies.

I advise young aggressive borrowers that it is easy to get into trouble, but extremely difficult to get out of trouble. Each of us has our needs and wants. The smart borrower addresses his needs first; a reckless borrower goes straight to his wants.

This is simple common sense, but in our world, common sense can be uncommon. Some young borrowers are under the impression that because they have no redeemable assets, a lender cannot hurt them in any way if they default. But that is not true. In the long run, a bad credit rating can destroy opportunity and make you a slave.

I consider all irresponsible aggressive borrowers as noncompulsive reckless gamblers with a penchant for spending beyond their means.

A few years ago, a twenty-nine-year-old woman sought my help to get over her compulsion to buy anything and everything in sight, whenever and wherever she could. Jennifer was the daughter of a wealthy businessman. At the time she came to see me, she was unemployed and had dropped out of college after two years. I asked her why she dropped out. She replied that she did not like the college environment or her professors. She had spent the last five years figuring out which college to switch to. One does not even need a high school diploma to figure out that she was irresponsible, impulsive, and spoiled.

I knew Jennifer's father well. He had come to see me to stop smoking and grinding his teeth in his sleep. I was able to help him on both counts. He told me that his daughter had always been a difficult child. She rebelled against any authority and discipline from a young age. She always made a fuss about everything. She was defiant about cleaning up her room, going to school, eating properly, and going to bed on time. Until their daughter was twelve, Jennifer's parents thought that if they bought her lots of toys she would appreciate them and cooperate. At times, this trick worked, but only for short periods. But once Jennifer became a teenager, no ploy was effective. She would bring home the most objectionable boys to meet her parents, and when her mother and father disapproved, she'd throw a tantrum and storm out of the house.

When Jennifer dropped out of college, her father asked her to work for him. He wanted to keep a close watch on her, and he hoped she would learn a sense of responsibility. But her spending sprees and reckless behavior only got worse.

Once she turned eighteen, Jennifer secured several credit cards. Every time she was mad at her parents or upset about something, she would go on a buying binge. Many times, the credit card bills would amount to $10,000 to $15,000 a month. She admitted that she sometimes accumulated debt just to irritate her mother and embarrass her father.

For some time, her parents tolerated these shenanigans. They'd give her stern lectures but eventually would pay her debts. But finally enough was enough. They told Jennifer she had to clean up her act. They would no longer be responsible for her debts. Her father sent her to me to see if I could help Jennifer turn herself around.

As I sat across the desk from Jennifer, I saw a young woman who had lost her grip on reality. She slumped sullenly in her seat, the chip on her shoulder as big as a house. How would I reach her and help pull her back into the world? How would I help Jennifer realize the possibilities that were within her reach? She was intelligent and beautiful, and she had parents who loved her and would do anything to see her succeed. She had it all, but she thought she had nothing.

I asked Jennifer to explain the situation from her perspective. She said that she loved her parents very much, but they didn't love or respect her. If they did, they would not treat her like a child. "They don't trust me, Dr. Prasad, but they tell me they love me," she said. "Where's the logic in that?"

Jennifer was hung up on respect, but she didn't understand it. She thought respect was her birthright, independent of her behavior.

"You can only command respect, not demand it," I said. I gave Jennifer a very strong lecture that day, and it was clear no one had ever spoken to her this way before. Her parents had been tiptoeing around her all of her life, fearful of her anger. They didn't want Jennifer to hate them, so they coddled her. In my office, the coddling ended.

"You're pissed off because the world isn't the way you want it to be," I said. "You want to ignore all the rules and do whatever you please, and you expect people to respect you. It's not going to happen. If you don't come down from your high horse, you won't make it. Maybe your parents will bail you out when things get bad, but one day, sooner or later, you'll be on your own and you won't have the resources—internal or external—to fend for yourself. Is that the future you want to envision?"

Jennifer was crying by now. I could see she felt bombarded by the truth. I had hit a nerve.

"Do you want to know how you can command respect?" I asked.

"Yes," she said, through her tears.

"Go get a job on your own. Move out of your parents' house, even if you can only afford a small place. Pay your own way. Right now you are a slave. Take back your life and decide what your future will be."

Jennifer did change her ways, although it took some time. I'm not implying that it was easy. There is no magic pill that can pull a person out of such a deep hole. But the truth is forceful, and my words made an impact on Jennifer because they reached her emotional core. It was as if she had been living in a dream, and now she was wide-awake.

Six years later, she came to see me, and she was a confident, smiling young woman. She had found her passion in jewelry making and had been moderately successful with her designs. She worked for an established jeweler and was hoping to go out on her own. The previous year she had married, and she and her husband were expecting their first child.

"I have one credit card to my name," Jennifer told me. "I only use it for convenience, and I never take it out if I don't have money in the bank to cover it. My husband says I'm a penny-pincher." She laughed. "I don't mind that title at all!"

When I treat young people who are trapped in the cycle of reckless spending, my thoughts often go back to my own youth. When my wife, Vashanta, and I were married, we barely had enough money to make ends meet, but my expectations were very high. We had moved to England from India with big hopes. I was planning to pursue a bright future as a cardiologist.

Several months passed, and I was unable to secure a residency in cardiology or in any other specialty. I was beginning to think I would have to return to India in shame when I was accepted for a residency program in psychiatry. It was one week before our first wedding anniversary.

I was tempted to buy an expensive anniversary gift for Vashanta, but deep down I knew I could not afford it. I weighed my options. Of course, I could have obtained a loan or bought the gift on installments at three times the prevailing interest rate. But my future was still uncertain, and I knew that a debt would weigh on me and distract me. On the other hand, I imagined how Vashanta's eyes would light up when I presented her with a lovely necklace. I wanted to be a big man—that successful doctor who could shower his wife with jewels. It was tempting.

Fortunately, I kept my priorities straight, and I played it safe by buying a pretty, but inexpensive, leather purse as an anniversary gift. On the day of our anniversary, when I presented the gift to Vashanta, she was so happy that I even remembered our anniversary in the midst of all my stress, that tears began rolling down her cheeks. She didn't care about the gift, only that I had thought of her. She actually wanted to return the purse to the store, because $20 was too much money. I insisted that she keep it. Even now, thirty-six years later, Vashanta protects that purse as if it were a million-dollar solitaire diamond. Since then, I have given her many expensive gifts, but the $20 purse is still her most precious and prized possession.

The Will to Change

Most of my patients are reasonably disciplined, productive, and sensible individuals. They recognize that they have a problem and are willing to correct it. If they could have done it on their own, they would have. But they were smart enough to realize that they needed outside help. However, not every compulsive gambler falls into this category.

Recently in the news, there was the story of a forty-four-year-old man who was convicted of burglary in the New York metropolitan area. This guy had robbed close to $2 million from about one hundred homes over the past two years. The thief was feeding his compulsive gambling habit through robbery. At night he would pick a home in a wealthy section and rob it to support his casino gambling habit. He loved to play several types of card games at the Atlantic City casinos. I was struck by his response when he was asked whether he regretted his actions. He said he didn't really see anything wrong with what he'd done. Such individuals don't think that it is fair for people to live in big, elaborate homes with expensive furniture, decor, jewelry, and equipment, while they themselves are forced to do hard labor just to make ends meet. They cannot find logic in this disparity. In their own way, they are equalizing what they consider the unfair distribution of wealth in society. They are like the bank robber who, when asked by a judge why he robbed banks, replied, "Because that's where the money is."

Lust for power, prestige, privilege, and wealth is not indigenous to underprivileged, uneducated street thugs. It is equally prevalent among the educated upper echelon of society. For example, I consider the junk bond king Michael Milken and many top executives from companies like Enron, Fannie Mae, and WorldCom to be greedy, compulsive, reckless gamblers. They are truly addicted to lavish lifestyles and the power to control the destinies of others. These savvy, sleek, devious, coldhearted crooks are the worst kind of compulsive, reckless gamblers. First, they are educated and intelligent and should know better; second, using sophisticated modern technology and twisted mathematical logic, they believe that they can control the future; third, they operate with impunity—they believe they are never wrong and it is everyone else's fault that the results did not pan out as planned. These individuals always gamble with other people's money, rarely their own. They have hurt thousands, sometimes millions, of people who believed in them. It is extremely difficult to rehabilitate this kind of compulsive gambler. Even time in jail and years of therapy leave them cold.

If you have a gambling problem, the first step in your recovery is finding the will to change. This means reaching inside yourself and acknowledging with humility that you have failed yourself and others through your actions. But it also requires a commitment to do what is necessary to reclaim your freedom. The program I have devised will start you on that path.

Part Two

The Prasad Method:
Mind over Habit

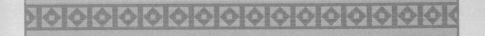

THE PROCESS OF overcoming a gambling addiction is not for the faint of heart. There's no such thing as a magic fix. Life isn't easy, and it isn't supposed to be. I often have patients complain, "It wasn't supposed to be this way." Well, who said so? All you have to do is look at human history to know that life is a battleground, not a playground. The truth is, we are still struggling every day for our survival, just like our ancestors. Even with the best planning and most conscientious effort, things don't always work out as we wish. However, we do have a lot of control over the quality of our lives and the way we choose to use our God-given talents and opportunities during our short stay on earth. To stop gambling recklessly and compulsively, you must take personal responsibility for your plight, and reject excuses and the sense of victimization.

It's not enough to know that your gambling habit is bad for you. You must believe it in your heart and soul. The fact is, people act on what they *believe*, not what they *know*.

The difference between what you know and what you believe is the real disparity between the action you should take and the action you do take. When we keep our ears open, we hear lots of sensible advice and compelling information. Why doesn't this information transfer to our beliefs? The information we hear has to pass through an emotional screen composed of our likes and dislikes. When we hear information that appeals to us, it receives easy passage. On the other hand, when we hear information that is not to our liking, it must pass through many more barriers. What we know for a fact is registered in the Intellectual Division. What we *believe* is registered in our Emotional Division.

I have never met a compulsive gambler who didn't want to get out of the terrible hole he had dug for himself. Every compulsive gambler knows that reckless betting is not in his best interest, but until this knowledge becomes a part of his belief system, any attempt to quit lacks real teeth. He may want to stop, but when push comes to shove he does not really want to part with the thrill he derives from games of chance, or with his high expectations for ultimate reward. A person's belief system must be altered in order to convince him to take actions that are not pleasing to him.

How do we know the truth? When it comes to beliefs, human beings are skillful at twisting the actual truth to their own version of the truth. We see this phenomenon all around us every day—in politics, advertising, business, and religious practices.

If you fight against nature's truth, you will lead a life of suffering. People say, "I love the truth . . . as long as it works out for me." Nature's truth is another matter. It is black-and-white. We want to negotiate the shades of gray. However, our excuses and explanations are all a waste of time. Nature doesn't care why you are taking outlandish risks. Nature sees only the action and passes judgment accordingly. Nature says only, "If you lose, you pay."

To stop your reckless gambling or spending habit, you must follow these steps:

Step 1: Understand Why You Must Stop. In order to successfully overcome a destructive habit, you must be uncomfortable with it. Obviously, as long as you are comfortable, you have little motivation to change. But something converts the comfortable habit into the uncomfortable habit—overwhelming debt, family problems, job loss, legal issues, and so on.

You must want to break the habit. You can no longer bear the idea of continuing. You may try to give up the habit but fail repeatedly. The desire to break the habit grows into a firm resolve or commitment to become permanently and happily free of it.

Step 2: Determine Your Depth of Addiction. The more information you have about your enemy, the easier it is to conquer. Knowing your own strengths and weaknesses will give you an edge in the manner of your response to the difficulties of quitting.

Step 3: Identify Your Addictive Profile. You must know why you are compelled to gamble or spend recklessly. What are the emotional triggers for your addiction? I have defined six primary addiction triggers: a sense of deprivation, entitlement, invincibility, disenchantment, insecurity, and defiance. The Addictive Profile, which is formed by one or more of these drives, is the engine that charges up addictive behavior.

Step 4: Make the Break. Don't tiptoe up to the line of stopping. Armed with a clear understanding of your habit and the tools to defeat it, you can end it for good. The Prasad Method enables you to pool all your strength to inflict a mortal blow against your enemy in a single stroke.

Step 5: Become a Responsible Gambler: Your final goal should be to change from being a reckless, compulsive gambler into a responsible gambler—a person who is able to handle the risks of life in a balanced manner.

Step 6: Live Your Life to the Fullest. You bring closure to the habit and move on to lead a life happily free of its constraints.

STEP 1

Understand Why You Must Stop Gambling

THE FIRST QUESTION I ask people who come to me to stop any addictive behavior is this: "Why have you decided to launch a personal vendetta against your beloved friend and companion?" That gets their attention!

I admire the people who come to my office with a hope of leaving a destructive addiction behind. They usually arrive filled with enthusiasm and determination to complete their missions. In buoyant voices, they talk about how eager they are to improve their lives, to break the chains of their harmful addictions, to start over with a clean slate. However, I am only interested in the reason that has firmly captivated their attention and compelled them to take action. I want to know about the force that drives them to forsake their old friend and companion—be it a slot machine, a glass of booze, or a cigarette. It takes a powerful motivation to succeed at this challenge. That motivation must come from within, and it must withstand the test of time.

Discovering Your Moment of Truth: An Inside-Out Approach

The following process is a variation of the one I use with my patients to help them realize their moment of truth and come to their own understanding of why they must stop their reckless gambling. It is designed to help you literally *change your mind* about gambling. By coming to the realization of why you really need to quit and understanding why you started gambling in the first place, you can make up your mind to put your habit behind you.

Coercion, even to advance a noble cause, never works as a solution. If guilt is the driving force, there is no chance that people will permanently give up the habit. The only effective motivation is an internal, voluntary desire to protect and preserve your quality of life by eliminating the destructive addiction.

Addiction is not an external reality, but an internal one, which must be viewed from the inside out. Unless you fully understand yourself and your motivations, you have no hope of permanently releasing yourself from the habit. If you've tried to overcome your habit before, only to fail, this time you'll start from an entirely different place. Instead of trying to wrestle the habit to the ground and kill it, begin by ignoring the gambling activity altogether. Focus instead on yourself. No two addicts are alike. Their temperament, outlook, attitude, priorities, expectations, and limitations are different from those of every other addict. For this reason, only *you* can break your habit. Not your doctor, not a pill, not your husband, not a therapist or support group. Just you.

The hardships you are encountering are mainly due to your own choices. You're responsible for your predicament, and you must spearhead the campaign to save yourself. This job cannot be delegated.

The chart on page 75 shows the difference between an inside-out approach and an outside-in approach.

Evaluate Your Reasons for Quitting

Sit down and seriously think about all the reasons you have for stopping your gambling or spending activities. Place each of the reasons you want to quit gambling into either the External box or the Internal box in the blank table on the following page. Calculate your score at the end. It will become part of your total Gambling Cessation Struggle Index—that is, the relative difficulty you will have in breaking the habit.

EXTERNAL REASONS INCLUDE:
- My wife has threatened to leave me if I don't stop gambling.
- The bill collectors are like hounds at my door.
- I'm a pariah with my friends.
- My work is suffering and I'm in danger of getting fired.
- I want to impress others.
- I want to set an example for my children.

INTERNAL REASONS INCLUDE:

- I believe gambling is not in my best interest.
- I want to have this monkey off my back.
- I want to feel good about myself and believe in myself.
- I will no longer be a slave to this habit.

EXTERNAL REASONS TO QUIT	INTERNAL REASONS TO QUIT
1. _____	1. _____
2. _____	2. _____
3. _____	3. _____
4. _____	4. _____
5. _____	5. _____

Score: For each External reason, give yourself 4 points. For each Internal reason, give yourself −1 point.
Total your score: _____
Enter the result in the Gambling Cessation Struggle Index calculator on page 99.

THE RIGHT WAY: THE INSIDE-OUT APPROACH	THE WRONG WAY: THE OUTSIDE-IN APPROACH
Don't talk. Commit yourself.	Keep talking about giving up gambling. Say you "would like" to quit.
Don't try to stop. Just stop.	Promise to give it a good try.
Believe reckless gambling is not good for you.	Believe you can go on a gambling spree every once in a while without doing damage.
Stop gambling for yourself—to improve your quality of life.	Decide to stop to please your spouse or boss.
Rely on your patience, tolerance, and strength to defeat the discomfort.	Rely on the antidepressants or other crutches to help you get by.
Make it your goal to put your gambling activity out of mind, not just out of sight.	Cut back on the amount of time or money you invest in gambling, instead of stopping altogether.

Determine Your Depth
of Addiction

NOT ALL reckless, compulsive gamblers will be successful in breaking the habit, and some will have a harder time than others. Where do you stand? Take the following test to determine the level of difficulty required to help you overcome your addiction. Read the following descriptions, then circle the numbers on the Depth of Addiction Meter, page 83, that apply to you.

The Age You Started Gambling

The younger the age when you start gambling, the stronger the imprint of the habit in the Emotional Division of your mind, making it much harder to give up. If you started gambling in your early teens or younger, it will be especially difficult to quit. You may not really remember a time when you didn't gamble. The activity is hard to separate from your identity.

Furthermore, studies have shown that adolescents who become heavy gamblers tend to have very strong emotional connections to the activity. They are less interested in winning big than they are in soothing anxiety, relieving depression, or building their self-image. Because they fail to learn healthy ways of handling their problems, they are more likely to continue this negative reinforcement into adulthood.

Jeff, a twenty-five-year-old landscaping laborer, came to me for help with his gambling problem, but I could see immediately that he didn't really believe he could overcome it. When I asked him what he thought was behind his problem, he shrugged and said, "I'm just a screwup, I guess."

"Why do you say that?" I asked.

"Because that's what everyone has been telling me my whole life," he said. "And guess what? They're right. I try to get my act together, but I always blow it."

Jeff's essential story about himself was formed in childhood, and it had a firm hold on him. He expected to fail, anticipated failure. He believed his destructive behavior was inevitable. People like Jeff are particularly hard to help, as their negative self stories have been building for a lifetime, the way plaque builds up in arteries, eventually hardening into unmovable beliefs.

Your Gender

Many studies have shown men to be much more likely than women to develop gambling problems and to become pathological gamblers. Men tend to have higher impulsivity levels and more aggressive tendencies—both key to the gambling habit. They also tend to start gambling younger than women do, as many gambling opportunities take place around sporting events.

Women, on the other hand, are more likely to be reckless spenders. It is estimated that 90 percent of compulsive shoppers are women. They are more inclined to associate happiness with procurement and with adorning or enhancing outer appearance. Women also suffer more from depression, which is a factor in overspending.

A Family History of Gambling

As with alcoholism, heredity may play a role in the development of a gambling addiction. Have others in your family had gambling problems? Genetic predisposition may work in conjunction with the trait of impulsivity to make you more open to reckless behaviors like gambling. There may also have been a strong social conditioning if your family often gambled for recreation when you were growing up.

Carlos, a thirty-five-year-old actor who sought my help conquering his gambling habit, identified this factor in his first visit to my office. "Like father, like son," he said wryly. He recalled that when he was a child, his father participated in a weekly poker game with a group of male friends where the stakes were high. His mother was strongly opposed to poker, since they were struggling to make ends meet, but his father insisted that he worked hard and had a right to a little entertainment with his buddies.

Carlos vividly recalled an incident that occurred when he was seventeen and working at an after-school job to earn money for college. His father took him aside one night and said, "I need to borrow some money." It wasn't a request but an order. "I emptied out my savings account and handed him the money,"

Carlos said. "I knew I'd never get it back. The last thing he said to me was, 'Don't tell your mother.'"

Carlos couldn't believe that now he was the one hitting up friends and family for their hard-earned money in order to feed a gambling habit. He didn't realize that in spite of his negative experience as a teenager, the stronger pull was to model himself after the father he adored.

Number of Attempts to Quit

One peculiar feature of addictive habits is that the first attempt to quit is the easiest, and that's when you have the best chance of winning. Irrespective of the technique—joining Gamblers Anonymous, taking antidepressants, cognitive therapy—the first attempt will be the most successful. If you've tried to stop gambling before but have been unsuccessful, the urge to gamble will be a lot stronger, and you will have a tougher struggle to succeed the second time and thereafter. But having learned a valuable lesson from your failed attempts, in your subsequent endeavors you may have a tendency to finally end your gambling activities for the rest of your life. This certainly confirms that human beings appreciate the results only if they endure a certain amount of hardship.

The Influence of Other Habits

According to the Gambling Impact and Behavior Study, conducted for the National Gambling Impact Study Commission, 20 percent of pathological gamblers have been dependent on alcohol or drugs in their lifetime. In fact, many research studies have found evidence of coexisting alcohol and drug abuse among pathological gamblers. Many people use alcohol and/or drugs when they gamble, whether at a casino, a racetrack, or the neighborhood poker game. Gamblers also use drugs to stay awake and to reduce stress while gambling. New research shows that among adolescents who gamble, alcohol and drug use is particularly high.

If alcohol or drug use is a part of your gambling habit, you will have a much harder time stopping. I always tell my patients that they must give up their use of these substances before they can hope to tackle their gambling problem.

Your Frame of Mind

Don't underestimate the importance of timing. The timing of your attack on your gambling habit is extremely important. In life, timing is the essence of a winning strategy. A perfect example is the Allied invasion of Normandy—the final, all-out attack on Hitler and his forces. The Allied leaders invested their entire hope of winning the war in this crucial move. The field commanders were setting up the stage, whereas the commanding generals focused on picking the perfect time for the invasion. History has revealed that the combination of precise timing and perfect execution by the Western military alliances literally changed the tide of the war. The invasion of Normandy was the beginning of the end of Hitler's barbaric, brutal regime.

Likewise, the timing of your attack on your gambling habit calls for careful consideration. The popular concept among behavioral therapists is that no time is better than the present to take action against an addictive habit. In theory, it sounds right. But the cold light of reality presents a different picture. I am convinced that there is a tremendous advantage in a well-prepared, preemptive attack against the habit.

Unfortunately, by the time the compulsive gambler is forced to stop, he has already created a great deal of damage in his relationships and work life. The debt collectors are at the door. He is feeling about as stressed as a person can be. It will be extremely difficult to simultaneously end his habit and manage the stress of quitting.

When you are in a state of depression or distress, the primitive emotions demand adequate compensation by associating with a pleasure seeking device. The threat of losing a job or a breakdown of your marriage can rattle you and affect your composure. We all know this from experience, and it is foolish to ignore reality. It is likely that, feeling depressed and despondent, you will seek refuge in your old comfort instead of fighting the habit.

The more balance you have in your life, the greater your chance of success. However, life does not always cooperate by presenting the perfect timing. That's why my method includes exercises to reinforce your spirits as you confront your enemy.

The overall category of frame of mind also includes such factors as whether or not your gambling has led to criminal charges, the strength of your support system from family and friends, and your future prospects to restore financial and emotional stability.

Whether You Have a Criminal Record

If you have been prosecuted for criminal activities related to gambling or spending—such as tax fraud, theft, illegal betting, or insurance fraud—you know what it's like to feel truly desperate.

A criminal record is just one more weight on your back, making it more difficult to successfully quit gambling. Not only will you have to battle prejudice from others, you will have to fight your own tendency to despair and your feelings of shame.

Your Support System

By the time many pathological gamblers hit rock bottom, they have lost the support of friends and spouses. I see this time and again. Having the support of people who believe in you and are willing to help you overcome your addiction is a valuable gift. For this, the greatest fight of your life, you need allies.

Your Future Prospects

How many bridges have you burned pursuing your addiction? Can they be rebuilt? When you have options available in your work and your finances, you'll have an easier time resisting the pull of your addiction. If you have lost your job and are barely making it financially, the temptation for a quick fix will be very strong, and it will be more difficult for you to see gambling for the sinkhole it is.

Your Depth of Addiction Score

Refined, disciplined, and dignified human behavior is like a well-maintained, manicured garden where a handpicked collection of color-coordinated shrubs, floral plants, hedges, and trees grace the landscape. This dream garden is the result of pride, good imagination, and dedicated hard work. The same holds true for refined behavior. Addictive habits are the untended weeds and crabgrass in the garden of our behavior complex. The longer the duration of our neglect, the harder the ability to restore our behavior to acceptable standards. Recognizing the presence of a destructive, addictive habit in a person's life is the beginning of the end of that habit. And taming such a habit is the final frontier in the saga of an addictive habit.

The following Depth of Addiction score will help you evaluate your personal level of attachment to your habit. The stronger your attachment, the greater your difficulty in quitting.

The Depth of Addiction Meter

Circle the number in each category that applies to your habit

AGE YOU STARTED GAMBLING	Under 18	3
	18–25	1
	Over 25	0
YOUR GENDER	Male	1
	Female	0
FAMILY HISTORY OF GAMBLING	Excessive or pathological gambling present in family history	2
	Raised in a family that enjoys recreational gambling	1
	No family history of gambling	0

(continued)

PREVIOUS ATTEMPTS TO QUIT GAMBLING	More than 3 serious attempts	3
	1–3 serious attempts	2
	Never tried to quit	0
INFLUENCE OF OTHER HABITS (circle all that apply)	Often gamble while drinking alcohol	3
	Also smoke marijuana	3
	Take psychotropic medications	2
	Take anti-anxiety prescription medications	1
YOUR FRAME OF MIND	Extremely distressed over events or circumstances	3
	Mildly stressed	2
	Relatively comfortable	0
CRIMINAL RECORD	Have a criminal record associated with gambling	3
	No criminal record associated with gambling	0
SUPPORT SYSTEM	Cannot count on family, friends, or employers for support	3
	Have family, friends, or employers willing to help you	1
FUTURE PROSPECTS	Lost everything, deep in debt, unemployed	3
	Lost a considerable amount, deep in debt, but still employed	2
	Lost a considerable amount of money, but still employed and not in desperate financial shape	1

Total: Add up the circled numbers. This is your total score. Enter it here and in the Gambling Cessation Strugggle Index calculator on page 99.

Now that you have a clear picture of your habit and the power it exerts over you, you have taken the first step toward reasserting control over your life. Let's examine your underlying motivations for your reckless behavior—those invisible drives that form the emotional basis of your Addictive Profile.

STEP 3

Identify Your Addictive Profile

IN CHAPTER 2, I touched on the drives of the Addictive Profile. To be effective against the gambling habit, you must understand the internally generated drives that feed it. These drives include a sense of deprivation, entitlement, invincibility, disenchantment, insecurity, or defiance. The stress of one or more of them primes the craving to gamble. Think of the mind of a pathological gambler as an emotional pressure cooker, fed by one or more elements of the Addictive Profile. As the pressure builds, you experience a growing discomfort, exhibited by agitation, rage, sleeplessness, the inability to concentrate, and so on. You believe that this pressure can only be relieved by gambling. At some point, when the psychological pressure becomes unbearable, the desire to gamble turns into a ravaging craving to release the pressure.

These intense cravings are caused by an emotional need. That need comes from a deeply rooted misconception about why gambling is a beneficial activity. The emotional drive of these stories allows people to continue behaviors that the rational mind clearly acknowledges as destructive. These drives demand action in order to be satisfied. Often a person will have more than one. They trigger the Emotional Division to seek relief.

None of us is completely free of these drives. They are integral to human emotions and in a proper balance can even enhance our lives and motivate us to achieve. However, for an addict, one or more of these drives take on a pathological character. For example, the normal influence of the Insecurity Drive is necessary to keep you alert and vigilant, thus enabling you to survive. An overactive Insecurity Drive paralyzes you and impairs your ability to make decisions. It also fosters dependency by encouraging you to rely on an external crutch in the guise of your habit to get you through the day.

The Addictive Profile, which is formed by an imbalance in one or more of these drives, is the engine that charges up addictive behavior. In this section, we will examine the drives of the Addictive Profile more closely, showing how an imbalance of one or more drives helps to keep you addicted. Take the quiz that is provided for each drive to determine whether it is out of balance for you. The results of these quizzes will provide essential clues to the nature of your addiction. As you evaluate your score, pay special attention to the drives that pose the biggest problem for you. These are the areas where you will have to concentrate your efforts.

The Deprivation Drive

A healthy fear of deprivation can be a positive motivator in life. It's what gets you up in the morning and sends you off to work to provide for yourself and your family. But a reckless gambler's fear of deprivation is extreme, and it is directly related to the activity of gambling itself. Gambling fills the emptiness you feel inside; no other activity quite measures up.

Is your Deprivation Drive out of balance? Take the following quiz to determine whether it plays a significant role in your gambling habit.

QUIZ: YOUR DEPRIVATION QUOTIENT

Read the following statements. In the box, give yourself
1 point for each statement that you agree with,
and 0 if it doesn't describe you.

STATEMENT	VALUE
You often feel physically tired or "burned out," especially toward the end of the day.	
You feel as if others are better off than you.	
You feel you are being unfairly forced to change your behavior.	
You often wish you had more friends.	
You have problems forming lasting relationships.	
You are easily overwhelmed by ordinary challenges, such as a broken pipe, a failed recipe, or a traffic jam.	
You think others have more opportunities or are luckier than you.	

You dislike your job or the treatment you receive from your boss or colleagues.	
You wish you had a cooperative spouse.	
You have a low tolerence for emotional discomfort.	

Score: Total the numbers in the right-hand column. That is your deprivation quotient. If your score is 1–5, you have a relatively normal Deprivation Drive. If your score is more than 5, your Deprivation Drive is overactive, making it a factor in your gambling habit.

The Entitlement Drive

A balanced sense of entitlement is important to your self-esteem. It allows you to feel special and motivates you to take care of yourself because your life is worth something. However, when your sense of entitlement is out of balance, you feel an overwhelming sense that you should be rewarded for living.

The mantra of the Entitlement Drive is "I deserve it." You feel it is your birthright to have what others have or to surround yourself with only the best, even when you don't have the resources to afford a lavish lifestyle. This drive is especially strong among reckless spenders—the so-called "shopaholics." Many parents inadvertently foster the Entitlement Drive when they indulge their children with expensive toys, usually purchased on credit. The cry of "Everyone else has one" is hard for parents to resist. In adulthood, reckless spending is often fueled by a belief that if you work hard and play by the rules, you deserve to be rewarded. I often see this, especially with single men and women living beyond their means. After long hours at the office, they treat themselves to a shopping spree, an expensive restaurant meal, or a fabulous vacation. There's nothing wrong with any of that, but if you have to borrow recklessly to pay for it, you're gambling with your security and peace of mind.

In the real world, entitlement of this kind does not exist. Actions have consequences. Just because you think you're entitled to reduce stress by spending wildly or blowing your paycheck at a casino doesn't mean you'll magically acquire the rent money.

Is your Entitlement Drive out of balance? Take the following quiz to determine whether it plays a significant role in your gambling habit.

QUIZ: YOUR ENTITLEMENT QUOTIENT

Read the following statements. In the box, give yourself 1 point for each statement that you agree with, and 0 if it doesn't describe you.

STATEMENT	VALUE
You often think that you work harder than those around you, and if something is going to get done, you have to do it yourself.	
You feel entitled to kick back and take a break every so often.	
You think you're justified in not always following the rules.	
You often feel that others do not understand you.	

You believe that hard work and accomplishment should be rewarded in a tangible way.	
You tend to seek instant gratification.	
You consider yourself special.	
When you see something you want, you buy it.	
You feel justified in doing your own thing, even when others depend on you.	
You often feel that you deserve more.	

Score: Total the numbers in the right-hand column. That is your entitlement quotient. If your score is 1–5, you have a relatively normal Entitlement Drive. If your score is more than 5, your Entitlement Drive is overactive, making it a factor in your gambling habit.

The Invincibility Drive

No human being is invincible, but this drive can have a limited positive effect. It's the underlying sense of personal power that gives us courage in seemingly impossible situations. Out of balance, however, the Invincibility Drive is pure arrogance. Pathological gamblers believe they have special powers that others do not possess. Perhaps their sense of invincibility was originally fueled by early victories, but eventually they'll confront the reality that they are vulnerable.

The Invincibility Drive is often especially strong among reckless spenders because it puts blinders over your common sense. You ignore the reality that you are spending beyond your means, and are sure you'll find a way out of the mess when the bills come due. Maybe you've managed the juggle in the past and believe you can do it again. Reckless gambling or spending driven by a sense of invincibility is the most dangerous form of gambling.

Is your Invincibility Drive out of balance? Take the following quiz to determine whether it plays a significant role in your gambling habit.

QUIZ: YOUR INVINCIBILITY QUOTIENT

Read the following statements. In the box, give yourself 1 point for each statement that you agree with, and 0 if it doesn't describe you.

STATEMENT	VALUE
So far, you've experienced no real problems from your unproductive habits.	
You like to cite exceptions to the rule, such as smokers who live to be one hundred or gamblers who usually win.	
You think of yourself as exceptionally strong.	
You like to beat the odds—in sports and at work.	
You are not impressed with authority.	
You march to your own drummer.	
You believe risk taking gives you a performance edge.	

You are highly successful in your profession.	
You tend to drive very fast and aggressively, and tailgate and honk at other drivers.	
You have no patience for people who are inept.	

Score: Total the numbers in the right-hand column. That is your invincibility quotient. If your score is 1–5, you have a relatively normal Invincibility Drive. If your score is more than 5, your Invincibility Drive is overactive, making it a factor in your gambling habit.

The Disenchantment Drive

Disenchantment is a necessary part of being human. We all have disappointments in life, and if we keep these setbacks in perspective we can learn from them. However, disenchantment can spiral into a sense of overwhelming gloom—the feeling that life has robbed one of joy. The wider the disparity between one's expectations and the actual reality, the deeper the disenchantment. Many people who are diagnosed as clinically depressed are actually experiencing disenchantment. The Disenchantment Drive can play a role in the gambling addiction when depression triggers a heavy reliance on a crutch just to see one through the day. Gamblers whose habits are fed by the Disenchantment Drive are less likely to worry about the consequences.

The Disenchantment Drive is especially strong for the reckless spender. Your life has not turned out the way you wanted, and you feel bitter and unhappy. Disenchantment drives you to spend in order to fill the emptiness and soothe the unhappiness.

The action of spending provides a thrill; it is more important than what is actually purchased.

Is your Disenchantment Drive out of balance? Take the following quiz to determine whether it plays a significant role in your gambling habit.

QUIZ: YOUR DISENCHANTMENT QUOTIENT

Read the following statements. In the box, give yourself 1 point for each statement that you agree with, and 0 if it doesn't describe you.

STATEMENT	VALUE
You have not had the life you dreamed of.	
You consider yourself a romantic and you daydream a lot.	
You think others succeed because they have inside connections or special advantages.	
You spend a lot of time in solitary pursuits.	
You have been sexually molested by someone you know.	
You often drink to excess or use recreational drugs to give you an edge.	
You are highly creative but have trouble executing your ideas.	

You tend to have a fatalistic attitude—what will be, will be.	
You have been treated for depression.	
You often feel bored.	

Score: Total the numbers in the right-hand column. That is your disenchant-ment quotient. If your score is 1–5, you have a relatively normal Disenchant-ment Drive. If your score is more than 5, your Disenchantment Drive is overactive, making it a factor in your gambling habit.

The Insecurity Drive

The Insecurity Drive is the opposite of the Invincibility Drive. In proper balance, these two drives give you a realistic idea of your potential. Out of balance, the Insecurity Drive involves a lack of courage to face the uncertain future and a lack of confidence in one's ability to tackle the challenges of a harsh world. Pathological gamblers with an overactive Insecurity Drive do not feel able to achieve success or even financial stability through their own abilities and talents. The gambling activity is an escape hatch. Gambling is also primarily a solitary habit. Slot machines are not judgmental! In fact, when the machine is spilling out piles of quarters, the gambler may see it as a form of approval.

Is your Insecurity Drive out of balance? Take the following quiz to determine whether it plays a significant role in your gambling habit.

QUIZ: YOUR INSECURITY QUOTIENT

Read the following statements. In the box, give yourself
1 point for each statement that you agree with,
and 0 if it doesn't describe you.

STATEMENT	VALUE
You are nervous and filled with anxiety in social settings.	
You worry that others watch you and judge you lacking.	
You are terrified of making a mistake.	
You consider yourself less attractive and less stylish than others.	
You grew up in an environment where adults were overly critical of you.	
You often feel lonely.	
You have trouble forming lasting relationships.	
If a friend cancels a date or your spouse is in a bad mood, you tend to assume you did something wrong.	
You don't believe you have the strength to stop gambling.	
You frequently have nightmares and disturbed sleep patterns.	

Score: Total the numbers in the right-hand column. That is your insecurity quotient. If your score is 1–5, you have a relatively normal Insecurity Drive. If your score is more than 5, your Insecurity Drive is overactive, making it a factor in your gambling habit.

The Defiance Drive

We all need a little defiance in our lives. It's what distinguishes us from robots. However, defiance for its own sake can get us into trouble. Many times a reckless, compulsive gambler continues the activity as a gesture of defiance. The zeal of this drive is such that gamblers don't even worry about the consequences of their behavior or quality of life. They consistently downplay the risks or outright ignore them. In most cases the Defiance Drive is fueled by the Invincibility Drive.

The rebellious tendency is more pronounced in adolescents, but it usually softens as a person matures. Young rebels are likely to take up unproductive behaviors like reckless gambling or spending, and as they grow and become less adventurous, they may still retain traces of habits they acquired at an earlier age. In some cases, a person will become addicted to a habit that persists long after the rebellious urge has passed. In other cases, the rebellion is so deep that a person holds on to the habit, refusing to yield, in the belief that it represents the very core of his identity.

Occasionally, the Defiance Drive can coerce an individual to go on perpetual wild spending binges. An individual with such a drive operates with a chip on the shoulder and invariably is out to settle a score.

Is your Defiance Drive out of balance? Take the following quiz to determine whether it plays a significant role in your gambling habit.

QUIZ: YOUR DEFIANCE QUOTIENT

Read the following statements. In the box, give yourself
1 point for each statement that you agree with,
and 0 if it doesn't describe you.

STATEMENT	VALUE
You believe you were born to change the world for the better.	
Other people don't understand your good motives.	
You think you understand the true issues concerning human nature better than most people.	
Many people you come across are hypocrites.	
Powerful people don't care about the little guy.	
You love to lead others but hate to follow.	
You believe that sometimes the end justifies the means.	
You've always had a troubled relationship with your parents, authority figures, or other adults.	
You believe you are a true individual.	
You tend to have a short attention span and to be short-tempered.	

Score: Total the numbers in the right-hand column. That is your defiance quotient. If your score is 1–5, you have a relatively normal Defiance Drive. If your score is more than 5, your Defiance Drive is overactive, making it a factor in your gambling habit.

STEP 4

Make the Break

YOU'VE DONE YOUR RESEARCH, and you're now armed with a clear picture of who you are as a reckless gambler. Now it's time to use that information to establish a new identity as a responsible nongambler.

Calculate Your Gambling Cessation Struggle Index

Your scores in the previous sections will help you determine the difficulty of quitting and the potential pitfalls you face.

Write down your scores from the calculators in the previous section:

1. Reasons for Quitting: _____
2. Depth of Addiction Meter: _____
3. Addictive Profile: _____

Add the three numbers. This is your total score. Refer to the table below to determine how long you can expect to spend in each cessation grade.

INTERPRETATION OF THE POINTS

Total your points from the three sections. The higher the score, the harder it will be for you to break your habit.

Score of 40 or more	Very difficult to rehabilitate
Score between 25 and 39	Moderately difficult to rehabilitate
Score between 15 and 24	Slightly difficult to rehabilitate
Score of 14 or below	Easy to rehabilitate

If your score is 14 and below, you may be able to conquer your gambling habit on your own, using the process in this book. However, it is always helpful to have the support of a partner or close friends. If your score is 15–24, you might also be able to break your habit without professional help, but you will need strong support from family and friends. If such support is unavailable, you will need to seek professional help. If your score is 25–39, you will almost certainly need professional help, and if your score is 40 or above, that help may need to be long-term.

What You Face

More than any other addiction, compulsive gambling can be clearly understood as a problem of the mind. There is no chemical substance at work, no stick of tobacco to crush out, no glass of booze to pour down the drain. It's just you, the gambler, and your will to survive and prosper.

Many of my patients find this sheer nakedness frightening. I'm asking them to rely on their own inner resources in order to succeed, yet their weaknesses have got them into this mess in the first place. By the time they come to me, they are models of poor self-esteem, crushing doubt, shame, and despair. They can't imagine how they can help themselves. I tell them to take it one step at a time.

State your commitment in irrevocable terms. Don't say, "I'd like to quit gambling," or "I'll try to quit gambling." This is not a commitment, only a wish. There is a big difference between wishful thinking and commitment. Wishful thinking causes you to give it a good try; when you fail, you will then say, "Better luck next time." When there is true commitment, failure is not an option.

Think of it as a contract you are making with yourself that has no escape clause. To be successful, the contract must include:

- A decision to tackle the habit on its terms and conditions, not those you imagine or invent
- A decision that failure is not an option
- A decision to be not just free of the habit but *comfortable* and *productive* without the habit
- A decision that you, not your habit, will decide your fate

If you're ready to stop gambling, but are afraid of your enemy and feel almost certain that you'll fail in its presence, you've lost the battle before you've even begun. Conversely, if you have taken an inside-out approach, and are ready to put your reckless behavior squarely in the past, you will win the battle.

STEP 5

Become a Responsible Gambler

RON, THIRTY-NINE, was desperate to get off the perpetual roller-coaster ride of betting, losing, and betting again with no end in sight. But the issue was far deeper and more complex than he had imagined. When he came to me for help, I advised him that it was not enough for him to just stop betting on the games. That was only half the battle. The full battle was to change his outlook, attitude, values, and priorities—to discover how to lead a peaceful, meaningful, productive, and memorable life. In order to achieve this, Ron had to harness his strength and overcome his weaknesses, meaning he had to tackle his perpetual reckless betting habit from a point of strength, not a point of weakness. "The question," I said, "is what makes Ron tick? What is going on inside your mind?"

Like many compulsive, reckless gamblers, Ron had never stopped to take a measure of himself and his life. But I immediately detected some clues. As he told me his story, I studied his face carefully. Sometimes facial expressions tell me more than words.

I noticed that when Ron spoke about his wife, Martha, his face became tense and his eyes grew cold. Even though he said that he loved his wife, his facial expression told another story. I guessed the reason.

Martha was angry and fed up with his habit. She was Ron's harsh judge, and she had threatened to leave him if he didn't get help. No man likes an ultimatum, even when it is stated with the best of intentions. Ron knew he had it coming, but he was still bitter. Besides the ultimatum, for the last two years the marital relationship had been strained because of financial woes and Ron's mental disposition. I knew then and there that this situation had to be rectified for several reasons. First, peace of mind is very important to recovery. Without peace of mind, Ron would surely fail. He was angry with himself, and could not see straight. He needed a staunch ally in his battle against his addiction. In my opinion, that would be his wife. She had stuck with him all these years.

When I shared my observations with Ron, he admitted that he was very angry with Martha. He felt that she should have been more sympathetic to his struggle. Instead, she was threatening to throw him out of the house. He thought it was unfair. He needed her cooperation, not her confrontation. I let him vent his anger; then I asked, "What would you have done if you were in her shoes?"

For a few seconds he was silent; then he said quietly, "I would have changed the locks and hired a divorce attorney." He dropped his head, momentarily stunned by his own admission.

"I believe your wife loves you or she wouldn't have stuck it out all of these years," I said. "Probably she feels more helpless in this situation than you do. She wants to help you, so she has given you the shock treatment in the form of a threat to shake up your jumbled mind. She is your best and only friend at this moment—don't lose her."

When I finished speaking, Ron had tears in his eyes. "I don't want to lose my wife," he said. "I am a religious man, Dr. Prasad. I want to do the right thing."

I was interested in Ron's claim to be a religious man. What did that mean to him? He explained that he was a staunch Catholic, who faithfully attended mass every Sunday. "And I pray for God's help every day of my life," he said with conviction.

"Yet you are spiritually deprived," I said.

Ron seemed offended by this. People do not like to have their religious dedication challenged, and even most therapists are reluctant to speak as boldly as I did. But I felt it was important for Ron to see a connection between his beliefs and his actions.

"You are selfish," I said. "You are blowing your money on bets and depriving your family of its security. Attending church religiously has not changed you for the better."

Ron hung his head. He knew I was right. But it wasn't my intention to further demoralize Ron. On the contrary, my aim was to lift his spirits and help him to get grounded. I viewed Ron as a drifter, with no clear direction in life. "Our destiny is like a house," I told him. "If you don't anchor the house firmly to the ground and build a solid foundation, it is only a question of time and wind speed before your house is blown away. The only way to secure your destiny in an unpredictable environment and an imperfect world is to shore up your foundation and anchor it to reality. The laws of nature accept no excuses. If you act like a drifter, you will be one in due course. It is cut-and-dried: survive or perish. It is your choice. Which will it be?"

I help my patients move toward a fuller understanding of self.

Your identity should not be based on external features and behaviors, such as skin color, clothing style, profession, zip code, the type of food you eat, club memberships, the language you speak, house of worship, whether you drink alcohol, whether you smoke, and the like. These factors are shallow. They may show style but they offer no substance to a well-formed sense of identity. When you rely on external factors, you are actually allowing the world to define you instead of taking a stand on your own. On the other hand, if you try to define yourself based on sound internal factors—your values, talents, priorities, temperament, expectations, tolerance, and life goals—you set yourself on a noble path. You become determined to reach your goals, even if it's hard. You can focus on the journey of your life without being bothered by insignificant or unproductive distractions.

Don't be a stranger to yourself. Know what makes you tick, so you can tackle the world around you. You cannot delegate this job to others. If you allow others to help you understand yourself, you will only see yourself through their eyes. This is a do-it-yourself project.

I recommend that you take your journal and write your answers to the following questions. Do this in a private place and take plenty of time to consider your answers. Tackle one question at each session, over a period of days or weeks.

1. **What are your core values?** That is, what in life is truly important to you after you strip away the layers of cover? Core values are usually all-encompassing and nonspecific. They apply in any circumstance. For example, my own core values include these two—not doing harm to others, and not taking advantage of others.

2. **What are your priorities?** If you are addicted to gambling, you've lost sight of your true priorities. Your life has been, literally, a game of chance—of acting first and thinking later. Now you must examine your life and decide where your energies will be directed. For example, is it more important for you to have close relationships with your coworkers than to make lots of money? Are you a homebody or a traveler? Are you family-oriented or a careerist? Be honest with yourself, because this is where you will stake your claim to the future. Your relationships have undoubtedly suffered because of your addiction. If you make it a priority to restore them, decide how you are going to fulfill this promise to yourself.

3. **What engages your interest?** When I treat compulsive gamblers, they often make statements like, "I used to love the theater, but I haven't been in years." Or "I had season tickets during the baseball season, but I stopped going when I started going to casinos." Or "I used to think I was a talented painter, but it's been a long time since I've picked up a brush." There's a reason why some activities engage you while others don't. Try to reconnect with your passions. This will lift your spirits and give you the confidence of being true to yourself.

4. **What are your strengths?** You're probably not feeling very strong right now, but every person has unique strengths. These strengths will support you in your efforts. They may have been in hiding—it's time to bring them out of storage.

5. **What are your weaknesses?** This is not an opportunity to beat yourself up. Rather, taking a calm, objec-

tive look at your shortcomings is an important step in your recovery—especially if your gambling was fueled by the Invincibility Drive.

Clear Your Mind with Meditation

Keeping your mind strong and supple will help you transform yourself from a reckless gambler to a *responsible* gambler in life. It will also reduce your stress during the battle to quit. Meditation can help you summon your mind's healing energy, retrieve your mind from a war zone, and place it in a neutral zone.

The objective of meditation is more important than the steps you take to get there. Meditating is not about disconnecting from the world around you. It is not about shutting off your five senses and making your mind passive in order to reduce stress. This won't work. Combatting stress requires clarity and the presence of your senses. Meditation helps you become centered within your reality; it is not an escape.

Meditation involves stepping back from the world for a short period. While you turn off your five senses, you must turn on the internal state that connects you with nature through your instincts. Meditation is not a passive state of mind. On the contrary, your mind will be in its most active state—more authentically than ever. Connecting with nature involves understanding its mandates about life and accepting its truth about your place in the world. This is both an exhilarating and humbling experience.

Every time I meditate I pick one or two issues in my life and strive to understand the full truth about them—not only how I perceive them but also nature's truth. Only then can I resolve the issues. This practice is relevant to the gambler. Not only must you consider your perspective, you must also strive to discover nature's truth—that if you continue to gamble you will suffer consequences. Accepting nature's truth will help you rise above the discomfort involved in quitting and embrace your full potential.

Meditation is a tool that can alleviate stress and strengthen your sense of purpose and will. But the process is not magical. You have to be open to seeing life as it really is, not as you want it to be. You have to choose priorities that elevate you, as opposed to the deceitful and destructive priorities you once held.

EXERCISE: VISUALIZE YOURSELF AT PEACE AND IN CONTROL

Sit in a comfortable position. Allow your arms to rest at your sides, palms up. Inhale and exhale slowly and deeply, keeping your eyes closed. Focus on the rhythm of your breathing and the movement of your abdomen and lungs as the healing energy flows through your body. Visualize your anxiety like a bird, and watch it fly away as you breathe in and out. Continue for at least five minutes or until you feel relaxed.

FREQUENCY AND DURATION

In the beginning, meditating once a day is enough. However, over the years the strong, positive mental high will become second nature. Eventually, even a brief meditation each day will keep you in good spirits throughout the day and allow you to face what comes your way as a challenge, not a chore.

TIME OF DAY

Find a time when you can comfortably spare thirty minutes or so without interruption. It can be any time of day. For me, early morning is best. I like to pool my energy and strength before I leap into the day's tasks.

LOCATION

Find a place without distraction—a quiet room in your home, a nearby park, or even a parking space in an empty shopping mall lot. Don't carry your cell phone or beeper. A small Walkman or MP3 player with appealing music is fine.

Strengthen Your Mind Through Nutrition

You may be surprised to find nutrition advice in a book about gambling addictions. However, most addicts, including compulsive gamblers, shortchange themselves nutritionally. They don't think about what they're eating, and they drink too much alcohol and coffee. I don't think I've ever met a compulsive gambler who was nutritionally fit. But it is impossible to have a clear and focused mind if you don't feed it with the proper nutrients. For this reason, I always include a nutritional component in my plan for compulsive gamblers.

Follow this regimen for two months to clear your mind and body:

1. Completely eliminate alcohol. You may not consider yourself an alcoholic, but alcohol is a depressant; it fogs the mind and contributes to a sense of helplessness and despair. Alcohol has also been associated with the gambling habit. Your battered neurons need to be regenerated so you can think with a clear mind.

2. If you drink coffee, replace it with green tea, which has a small amount of caffeine and also contains many beneficial antioxidants. Studies show that it is helpful in sharpening mental acuity.

3. Include protein in your first meal of the day. Protein increases energy, while heavy carbohydrates slow you down.

4. Avoid sugary, high-calorie snacks. Prepare snacks of raw fruits and vegetables or a handful of nuts. For an energy boost, make a shake of soy milk or yogurt and fresh fruit.

5. Limit red meat to three times a week, and keep your portion size to six ounces or less.

6. Limit wheat products to one serving per day.

7. Drink plenty of water—at least six to eight glasses a day.

8. Begin to exercise for at least thirty minutes every day, preferably in the morning. Exercise generates natural antidepressants (endorphins) that will improve your disposition and elevate your mood.

9. Keep a journal detailing what you eat, how much you consume, when you eat, and how you feel.

Check Your Expectations

Compulsive gambling is a problem of expectations. The idea of expectations is often misunderstood. High expectations are usually considered a positive thing—a form of optimism—but high expectations can also pave the way for disappointment and dampen the spirit. I am not saying that low expectations are preferable. The key is to have realistic expectations.

A good way to keep your expectations in check is to measure your worth by your performance, not the results. You can't always control the results, but you can control your actions. Once you identify your goal, decide the steps you need to take to fulfill that goal, then focus on them like a laser beam. Have the courage to accept the result, whatever it may be. If the result is to your liking, you can feel good about it. Conversely, if the result is not to your liking, don't let your world come to a standstill. Learn the lesson from your experience and move on. As long as you direct your expectations to your performance, you have nothing to fear and your spirits are never affected.

Let me give you an example of how one's performance can be affected by focusing on the results, not on the actions. One day I got a call from a former patient with a very strange request. Sam, a forty-seven-year-old lawyer, wanted me to help him with his golf game. "My handicap is twelve, but I know I can do better," he said. "Something is blocking me."

I laughed. "Sam, I don't even know what a handicap of twelve is. I know nothing about golf. How can I help you?"

Sam kept urging me, and I was intrigued, so I agreed to do what I could. I figured that if I failed to help him, the worst thing that would happen was that his golf game would stay the same, and that would not be the end of the world.

We didn't meet on the golf course, but in my office. After all, I wasn't a golf coach; Sam's problem was in his mind, not in his swing.

Sam told me that his handicap would go as high as ten to thirteen during important games at his golf club, but it would drop down to five or six during regular games, or when he played alone.

This did not surprise me in the least. Sam was a proud man, and he always tried to protect his image. Even in a friendly game of golf, where the wager could be as simple as a restaurant meal, he hated to lose. When he played in a tournament, he really got worked up. He became very anxious about the end result, and focused on the end rather than on the activity of playing. Naturally, the quality of his game suffered.

"Here is the answer to your problem," I told Sam. "Don't think about winning or losing. Just play the game." It sounded trite when I said it, but it was so true! "Don't let pride make a fool of you," I added.

Sam had to train himself to be less self-conscious, even in a friendly environment. He had to stop worrying so much about what others thought of him. This may seem easier said than done, since the world judges people by their results, not by their actions. But I assured Sam that if he concentrated on playing to the best of his ability, and was willing to accept the end result with good grace, his game would improve. A year later, Sam called to tell me that he was the number-one player at his club.

Restore Your Relationships

It is impossible to recover from your gambling addiction if your important relationships are in tatters, yet that is often the state gambling addicts find themselves in. A key to your recovery involves making amends. That means, first of all, that you must repay your debts—whether they be to friends, family members, or credit card companies. I assure you, this act alone will go a long way toward demonstrating your intention to change. After you have taken this first step, begin to slowly rebuild the relationships that you still have. Acknowledge the fact that you, and you alone, are responsible for the hurt you have caused.

RECKLESS GAMBLERS DEVASTATE FAMILIES

Like all addicts, reckless, compulsive gamblers devastate the lives of those who love them. A few years ago I treated Rena, a forty-two-year-old divorced working mother of two. Rena was suffering from depression since the breakup of her marriage. She wanted to feel good about life again, but she couldn't get past her ex-husband Steve's terrible betrayal. All you had to do was mention his name and her face would turn red and her nostrils flare with anger. "He betrayed my love, he gambled with our children's future, and he destroyed himself and us in the process," she told me. I asked Rena to tell me her story.

(continued)

Steve and Rena were married when they were both twenty-five. "He was my first true love," she said. Steve, who had a degree in chemical engineering, was full of ideas for their future. He was a real go-getter. Soon after they were married, Steve started an industrial dye business, and Rena worked for him for five years before their children were born. She was always very impressed by Steve's knowledge and the savvy way he interacted with customers. He was able to figure out the customers' needs the very first time he met with them, and he customized the product to fit their circumstances. In five years, the two built a successful and profitable business.

After that, Rena stayed home with the children, and Steve continued to run the business and build security for the family's future. But in due course he tasted the stock market. He had an excellent credit rating, and he started to bet on high-risk speculative stocks and bonds, hoping for high profits in a short period. Just like many other investors, he knew when to buy but he did not know when to sell. Greed and pride together make people lose their common sense and turn even a street-smart individual into a dumb, impulsive investor. He was completely lost in the quagmire of stocks and bond trading when he began to trade on margin accounts. Gradually, he neglected his business and sank deeper into debt.

Rena did not have a clue about any of this, but toward the end she noticed that Steve was agitated, short-tempered, and restless and had trouble sleeping. When she asked him what was bothering him, he would brush off her concerns and tell her it was just the usual business headaches and nothing to worry about. She realized something was really wrong when she started to get nasty phone calls from collection agencies. Finally, one day Steve left for work and never returned. Eventually, Rena learned the reason for his disappearance. He owed the IRS more than a million dollars in unpaid taxes.

Rena felt that her whole world had collapsed. She was dumbfounded, and had no idea how to sort out the mess her husband had left her. She declared bankruptcy, and lost everything. She and the children moved into a small rental apartment, Rena found a job as an office manager, and she put her dreams on hold as she struggled to get back on her feet.

Steve was not around to see the devastation he had caused, but gambling addicts need to face the terrible truth that their actions ruin the lives of those they love the most.

Tame the Future

We cannot have absolute certainty about what the future will bring. Even so, life demands that we take action. For all practical purposes, taking on a task means taming the future. Now that you have done your homework in the previous steps, you are ready to take on the tasks that will fulfill your goals and ambitions—be they reconnecting with friends, finding a life partner, starting a job, or getting involved in the community. Usually, it is better to take on one task at a time, especially if it is an important task.

Compulsive gamblers are accustomed to acting first and thinking later. Now you are required to do just the opposite. Do your homework. Break down the task to its simple components. Study each and every component in depth, and figure out how they fit into the complete puzzle. Be methodical. As you slowly rebuild your life, remember these important facts. They will give you strength:

- Understand that what's done is done. Take your gambling losses in stride and do not try to recover your losses. Your gambling days are over.
- Swallow your pride and approach your life with humility. It is not necessary for you to appear to be a big shot in front of your friends.
- Change your priorities from making money as number one. Making money goes on the list after freedom, peace of mind, and good health.
- Pay more attention to your family, and make an effort to give them gifts that are not material, but that require time, support, and affection.
- Stop fretting about what the world thinks of you. Focus on meeting your own highest standards, not theirs.

Eliminate the Mentality of Addiction

Addiction is a form of slavery, and the goal should be freedom. Unfortunately, the current culture of "recovery" promotes the idea of "once an addict, always an addict." Many of my patients tell me that their greatest desire is to be completely free of the compulsion to gamble or spend recklessly—to feel no tug of desire toward their old habit whatsoever. Is this possible?

This is where I part ways with the Twelve Step ideology, which many gambling recovery programs, such as Gamblers Anonymous, are now using. The Twelve Step method encourages gamblers to think of their addictions as permanent—like dormant bombs set to explode without warning. Constant vigilance is required. What a drag! In my experience, what addicts really long for is normalcy—the state of comfortable nonaddiction—not continued obsession. After all, their addiction has already stolen years from their lives When they look at themselves in the mirror, they don't want to say, "I am a compulsive gambler in recovery." Such a pronouncement can do little more than sap the spirit. Likewise, to say, "I am a former compulsive gambler" has a very different effect on the mind than to say, "I am not a reckless gambler," or "I am a responsible gambler." Mind you, this attitude is very different from that of complacency. You will always maintain a realistic view of yourself, but gambling will not be a constant monkey on your back.

Through the emotional adjustment, most people are able to control the desire to seek comfort from habits on a day-to-day basis. However, they almost always say they carry a deep dread of what will occur the first time they experience a highly stressful situation. They don't trust their instincts to choose a different, more productive method of relief—probably because they've "fallen off the wagon" so many times in the past.

If you are to be successful in conquering your enemy, you must face your habit without fear. That is possible with the inside-out approach. It is not possible with the outside-in approach.

Eliminating the mentality of addiction is the most crucial step in the process—the one that makes change permanent. How is it accomplished? Remember, the Instinctual Division of the mind is not independent of the Intellectual and Emotional divisions. The instinct to turn to gambling in times of stress is a learned behavior. Even when the Emotional Division is no longer demanding relief, the Instinctual Division must be reconfigured to respond differently. In essence, it must be trained to have an alternative automatic response to stress.

In essence, it is knowing the difference between truth and illusion when you decide what will make you happy or relieve your stress. My mother once gave me some invaluable advice. She said, "Son, stick with the absolute truth, and you will be a survivor. The truth is like a wildfire that no one can contain. It consumes everything around it. The truth is the last thing standing, after all the cowards and liars have run away. Align yourself with the truth, and you will stand with it."

Over the years, I have found my mother's advice to be reliable, and I have passed it along to my patients. It provides a lesson for those who approach life with cockiness, who delude themselves that they are above the laws of nature. Gamble we must, but the key is to live this gambling life in an honest, responsible way.

If you approach each of these six steps with full commitment and focus, I assure you it will be difficult, if not impossible, for you to return to your compulsive ways. One cannot be immersed in both illusion and reality at the same time!

STEP 6

Live Your Life to the Fullest

SINCE LIFE IS A GAMBLE, the ultimate goal of any compulsive gambler is to become a responsible gambler. What does a responsible gambler look like? The responsible gambler is well-balanced, with equal parts confidence and caution. He is assertive, but not arrogant. He is ambitious, but not greedy. He is patient, but not lazy. He is cool and calm, but not a coward. He does not hesitate to disagree with others, but his aim is not to insult or humiliate them. He backs up his words with action, and follows through on his commitments. He commands respect, but does not demand it. He usually keeps his eyes, ears, and mind open, and his mouth shut. He speaks little, but makes a lot of sense. Finally, he thinks first and acts later.

I know, it sounds good on paper, but could any human being measure up to all this? It's true that we all have flaws, but I have come across many people who have exhibited these traits in varying degrees. I'm not talking about extraordinary people, but ordinary folks like you and me. They're teachers, nurses, accountants, office managers, small-business owners, and blue-collar workers. They receive little in the way of public acclaim, but they go about their lives with integrity, and their qualities are well known to the people who love and admire them. The wonderful secret of humanity is that each of us has it in our power to be remarkable in our own life. Being human, at one time or another, we all make mistakes and fail to act in our best interests. The irony is that by virtue of our superior intelligence, humans are supposed to be the masters of logic. Often, lower animals exhibit more logic than we do. That's because they act according to their primary instincts. They lack the complex intellect and emotions that drive human behavior.

Even so, humans don't wish to exchange their fantastic gifts of intellect and emotion for a life on automatic pilot. These abilities make our lives worth living. We relish the unpredictability of our existence because it brings unlimited possibility. To be human is to gamble with the future every day. It's second nature to us. However, it can also destroy us. I believe that the thrill of an unpredictable outcome and our zeal to control the uncontrollable are the cornerstone of mind-provoking addictions, such as gambling.

The responsible gambler handles the uncertainties of life by accepting that he cannot have both excitement and security at the same time. This is a simple fact. The higher the security, the lower the degree of excitement. The lower the security, the higher the degree of excitement. We constantly shift between these two options while planning our activities. Whenever we lean toward the second option, we have opted for gambling chances instead of calculated chances. I believe that this component decides the intensity of the gambling streak in us. A responsible gambler, who focuses on security while betting on his odds to win, is a safe and smart gambler. But he has to sacrifice some of the thrill and excitement. Hence, a responsible gambler is not a passionate gambler.

The thrill of momentary uncertainty, with heightened hopes of winning, lures people toward gambling. If an individual can strike a balance between the excitement, logic, and hope without losing touch with reality, he will not succumb to the gambling fever.

It is not just the thrill that drives the gambling instinct. I believe that the element of hope is just as important. To get something for nothing has always been an attractive proposition for human beings. When we wager a dollar for a lottery ticket, we have the momentary fantasy of reaping an enormous financial gain, leading to unlimited control over our destiny, and total peace of mind. Unfortunately, there is anecdotal evidence from the confessions of many lottery winners who state that their lives did not turn out so well after they hit the jackpot. In some cases, their lives were ruined. Most people pay no attention to these stories, believing that *they* would manage their winnings differently. They say, "It's better to be rich and miserable than to be poor and miserable." What they don't recognize is the simple fact that people who enjoy reasonable peace, happiness, and contentment before they win the lottery will invariably retain their sense of well-being afterward as well, while discontented, angry, and unhappy people will most likely remain miserable whether they are rich or poor. Happiness and peace of mind cannot be purchased.

How can you make the change permanent, so that you literally lose the desire to gamble recklessly? Remember, the Instinctual Division of the mind is not independent of the Intellectual and Emotional divisions. The instinct to gamble recklessly in times of stress is a learned behavior. Even when the Emotional Division is no longer demanding the relief, the Instinctual Division must be reconfigured to respond differently. In essence, it must be trained to have an alternative response to stress.

How do you perform an instinctual reconfiguration that will change your automatic response to stress? How can you erect a permanent barrier against your enemy?

We all face obstacles in life regularly. Sometimes we are distressed, upset, disappointed, or hurt. Being treated unfairly by others hurts us the most. Believe it or not, it happens to us all the time. Pain and anguish demand immediate compensation. We need to do something to soothe the pain at that moment of distress. We take an inventory of what activities have given or could give us relief and comfort on such occasions. Usually, addictive habits are at the top of that list, and we go for them, even if we have once parted with them. Your task will be to evaluate the other items on that list that you can use instead.

I ask my patients to perform visualization exercises—to picture themselves at the final moment when they close the door on their gambling habit and lock it behind them. Some have difficulty looking ahead; some balk at locking the door. Some experience a sudden urge to take one last look. This exercise is immensely powerful. It completes the emotional adjustment. Closing the door, placing a sturdy lock on it, and throwing away the key, the individual bids a lasting farewell to the habit, with no possibility of returning. If all of the previous steps have been completed, this closure feels completely natural.

As you begin to see yourself and your place in the world in a more realistic light, these priorities will emerge naturally: peace of mind, unadulterated good health, freedom, and the natural high that comes from being at one with nature. When your priorities are straight, everything else falls into place. You may still strive to make good money, but the desire for money won't run you. You may seek material comforts, but not need them for your well-being. Your relationships will occur naturally on your own terms; you will no longer feel the need to create facades to make yourself more popular.

Here is another lesson from my wise mother. When I was an adolescent, she told me, "Don't ever chase after fame or fortune. You will become their slave."

I was a sassy young man, so I replied, "You have told me what *not to do,* but you haven't told me what *to do.*"

She smiled at me and replied, "Simple: keep your priorities straight and strong. Never try to compete with your fellow human beings, only with yourself. Bring the best you have to offer to every day, and let nature take its course. I promise you, if you do this, fame and fortune will chase after you but they will never own you. Instead, you will own them."

My mother's advice stayed with me. I wanted this freedom. It is one reason I do the work I do—to show others the way out of their slavery.

APPENDIX

Ask Dr. Prasad

Is it really possible to quit gambling following the method in this book? Don't people need hands-on treatment or support?

Obviously, reading a book is a bit different from seeking personal treatment. For those who are strongly motivated to quit gambling, and don't have large barriers, the book should be enough. Others may need more help. But I strongly believe that using the book to take your solitary journey is a good start. Remember, you alone can overcome your habit. Not a support group or a therapist. Just you.

Do you offer more than your philosophy and strategies to your patients?

Yes, I do. I guide my patients through two steps. First, all patients are exposed to the concepts I have outlined in this book. Many times that is sufficient for an individual to part with his habit. To complete this step, a patient will visit me from one to three times, depending on the number of drives that control his habit. Second, my patients receive special hands-on treatments, which I have devised to offer a head start for true, hard-core addicts who have lost confidence in their ability to give up their habits. Usually, this step takes two or three treatments over a period of ten to fifteen days. These treatments boost the patient's confidence, conviction, and level of tolerance of emotional discomfort, thereby allowing him to conquer his addiction.

I read that pathological gambling is caused by a chemical imbalance of neurotransmitters to the brain, and can be treated with antidepressants or anti-anxiety medications. What is your opinion?

It's true that there is a theory among some within my profession that the compulsion to gamble is caused by an imbalance of the neurotransmitters that control mood and regulate the pleasure centers in the brain. These include serotonin, norepinephrine, and dopamine. I disagree with this assessment of the problem. I do agree, however, that depression can be a factor in a gambling addiction. For some individuals, gambling becomes a form of self-medication when they feel lonely or dispirited. They gamble to boost their morale and inject some fun into their life. Unfortunately, what appears to work initially, usually fails in the long run.

The best way to approach the problem is through the mind, not the brain. However, I acknowledge that a small percentage of extremely entrenched addicts may need short-term help from anti-anxiety and antidepressant medications to recover from a gambling addiction. If you are one of these individuals, talk to your doctor about a prescription—but I encourage you to use the medication only for seven days.

How can compulsive gambling be a disease, when there are no biological symptoms?

I equate all addictions, including gambling, with cancer of the mind. The addiction corrupts the mind first, causing it to act against itself—similar to the way that cancer cells destroy healthy cells in the body. Eventually, the process leads to irrevocable damage.

Can a person who goes to a casino every weekend, but gambles only a set amount of money, be considered a responsible gambler?

A responsible gambler is balanced and sensible. It seems to me that gambling every weekend is like playing with firecrackers—it can be fun, but you have to be extremely vigilant not to cross the line of safety.

I advise people to restrict the number of times they visit casinos and to make the trip part of a larger recreational event that includes dining, sightseeing, going to shows, and such things. It is absolutely crucial to set aside a fixed dollar amount for these activities well in advance. Don't be tempted to extend that fixed amount, even by one dollar. If you do so, you have crossed the line.

A couple of times, my wife and I have played the slot machines in Atlantic City. Before we entered the casino, we fixed the dollar amount that we were going to spend, and kept on playing until we reached our limit. Once in Las Vegas, while we were playing a slot machine, Vashanta hit the jackpot and won $900. At that point, we'd lost $150 between the two of us. It was tempting to keep playing with our winnings, hoping for even larger rewards, but, knowing that the odds are fixed in favor of the casino, we decided to quit and take our $750 profit with us. Once we were outside the casino, we noticed how our adrenaline began to normalize. We took a deep breath and decided to go out for a nice dinner.

How can I make sure that my children do not get involved in gambling?

My mother often said, "There are many intelligent people in this world, but there are few smart people." Kids today must be smart to avoid a host of pressures— to use drugs, smoke, have sex, or drink alcohol. Increasingly, gambling is being added to the mix. As parents, you can play a crucial role in helping them to be smarter.

First, know that actions speak louder than words. If you gamble, even recreationally, your moral authority is zero. Many parents complain that their kids don't pay any attention to what they do or say. This is absolutely wrong. You are a more important influence on your children than their peers or all the forces of society they encounter outside the house.

Second, take an inside-out approach. You can lecture them about bad habits until kingdom come, but it will have little effect if the inner building blocks are not there. Help your children develop strong self-esteem and inner resolve so they won't become ruled by the Addictive Profiles. Teach them that happiness and a sense of purpose come from within—they are not given to them by others or achieved magically. Enable them to understand the blunt realities of nature—that if they make mistakes, nature issues consequences. Show them by your words and actions that a fulfilling, exuberant life can be achieved. When they see you living with joy, they will want to emulate you.

Do people who are down on their luck or struggling financially have a harder time breaking bad habits?

Not necessarily. The key is what's going on inside. My patients are often men and women of great privilege. They are wealthy, successful, the envy of their peers. They have it all. They are also people who are trapped by addictions—to gambling, smoking, alcohol, food, drugs, sex—or haunted by debilitating fears and phobias. In them, I observe the paradox of human behavior. On one hand, my patients are smart and powerful. On the other, they are foolish and destructive. They have won the lottery of life, yet they are disappointed. They have failed to take full measure of themselves—who they are and what is possible for them. Instead, most of them define themselves by the way the world treats them. This is the source of much suffering and wasted energy. They worry about deficiencies that only exist in the eyes of the world.

You are so passionate about your work. Where did you learn your philosophy? Did it evolve from your own experiences?

I am an ordinary human being, just like everyone else, and I wasn't always such a happy camper. I found my vision in my struggles. Let me tell you the experience that changed my life.

I was born in India, a country of deprivation, and yet I grew up in comfort. All my life I was treated like a prince. And so, when I left India to pursue a medical residency in England, I was full of arrogance. My attitude was, "I am doing you a great favor by coming here. You need me more than I need you. I am special."

When I arrived in England, with my young wife in tow, I expected the red carpet treatment. I applied to the top programs in neurosurgery and in cardiothoracic surgery—and one after the other, I was rejected. I was accepted into only one program, which was not the one I wanted. It was a psychiatry residency.

I was angry. I felt disillusioned, betrayed, lost. My first reaction was, "You can't treat me this way. I'm going home." But one night, hours before I was scheduled to leave, I had a realization. For the first time in my life I was confronted with a challenge, and what was my response? To run back to safety.

I took a hard look at myself: "Balasa, you think you are better than everyone else. You think you have something special to offer. You are not special. No one is special. Nature does not treat you like a special case. You need this world as much as this world needs you. Don't you forget that."

That night, I decided I would not run away. I would stay and fight. I signed up for the psychiatric residency.

My humiliation woke me up. I crashed into the absolute truth of Almighty Nature. Not the way I wished it would be. The way it was. Almighty Nature—or God, or whatever you call the great force of the universe—has its rules. It's up to us to figure them out. There are no free rides. No special circumstances. So I took what was available to me. But then I saw I had another choice to make. I could embrace the challenge fully or I could be halfhearted, bitching all the way. I chose. I said, "I am going to put my heart and soul into this psychiatric residency." And that is when I crossed the line between merely accepting my fate and using my fate to create my masterpiece. My work became exhilarating and fulfilling. It was not the ending point. It was the beginning point. In the coming years, I was able to build on my clinical training to give me insight into the mind and body from different perspectives. After completing a residency in psychiatry, I pursued residencies in internal medicine and family medicine to better grasp the association between body, mind, and behavior. When I moved to the United States in 1972, I took on a fourth residency in anesthesia, to study the influence of powerful analgesics, hypnotics, and tranquilizers. By the time I opened my practice in behavior modification, I had developed a system that integrated the Eastern wisdom of my heritage with the vast potential of Western technology.

I persevered in my profession because I learned the lesson of humility: *Ask not what the world can do for you. Ask what you can do for yourself.* Life presents an opportunity. Find out what you can do with it. I have found a way to be master of my destiny. I have found peace of mind, clarity of mission. My message to you is simple: if I can do it, so can you all.

INDEX